God's Waiting Room

Global Perspectives on Aging

Series editor
Sarah Lamb

This series publishes books that will deepen and expand our understanding of age, aging, ageism, and late life in the United States and beyond. The series focuses on anthropology while being open to ethnographically vivid and theoretically rich scholarship in related fields, including sociology, religion, cultural studies, social medicine, medical humanities, gender and sexuality studies, human development, critical and cultural gerontology, and age studies. Books will be aimed at students, scholars, and occasionally the general public.

Jason Danely, *Aging and Loss: Mourning and Maturity in Contemporary Japan*
Parin Dossa and Cati Coe, eds., *Transnational Aging and Reconfigurations of Kin Work*
Sarah Lamb, ed., *Successful Aging as a Contemporary Obsession: Global Perspectives*
Margaret Morganroth Gullette, *Ending Ageism, or How Not to Shoot Old People*
Ellyn Lem, *Gray Matters: Finding Meaning in the Stories of Later Life*
Michele Ruth Gamburd, *Linked Lives: Elder Care, Migration, and Kinship in Sri Lanka*
Yohko Tsuji, *Through Japanese Eyes: Thirty Years of Studying Aging in America*
Jessica C. Robbins, *Aging Nationally in Contemporary Poland: Memory, Kinship, and Personhood*
Rose K. Keimig, *Growing Old in a New China: Transitions in Elder Care*
Anna I. Corwin, *Embracing Age: How Catholic Nuns Became Models of Aging Well*
Molly George, *Aging in a Changing World: Older New Zealanders and Contemporary Multiculturalism*
Cati Coe, *Changes in Care: Aging, Migration, and Social Class in West Africa*
Megha Amrith, Victoria K. Sakti, and Dora Sampaio, eds., *Aspiring in Later Life: Movements across Time, Space, and Generations*
Cristina Douglas and Andrew Whitehouse, eds., *More-than-Human Aging: Animals, Robots, and Care in Later Life*
Casey Golomski, *God's Waiting Room: Racial Reckoning at Life's End*

God's Waiting Room

Racial Reckoning at Life's End

CASEY GOLOMSKI

RUTGERS UNIVERSITY PRESS
NEW BRUNSWICK, CAMDEN, AND NEWARK, NEW JERSEY
LONDON AND OXFORD

Rutgers University Press is a department of Rutgers, The State University of New Jersey, one of the leading public research universities in the nation. By publishing worldwide, it furthers the University's mission of dedication to excellence in teaching, scholarship, research, and clinical care.

Library of Congress Cataloging-in-Publication Data

Names: Golomski, Casey, author.

Title: God's waiting room : racial reckoning at life's end / Casey Golomski.

Description: New Brunswick, New Jersey : Rutgers University Press, [2025] | Series: Global perspectives on aging | Includes bibliographical references and index.

Identifiers: LCCN 2024012715 | ISBN 9781978840607 (paperback) | ISBN 9781978840614 (hardcover) | ISBN 9781978840621 (epub) | ISBN 9781978840638 (pdf)

Subjects: LCSH: Nurse and patient—South Africa. | Racism—Health aspects—South Africa. | Racism—South Africa. | Nurses, Black—South Africa. | Older white people—South Africa. | South Africa—Race relations.

Classification: LCC RT86.3 .G65 2025 | DDC 362.61089/00968—dc23/eng/20240820

LC record available at https://lccn.loc.gov/2024012715

A British Cataloging-in-Publication record for this book is available from the British Library.

Copyright © 2025 by Casey Golomski

All photos were created by the author with subjects' permission.

All rights reserved

No part of this book may be reproduced or utilized in any form or by any means, electronic or mechanical, or by any information storage and retrieval system, without written permission from the publisher. Please contact Rutgers University Press, 106 Somerset Street, New Brunswick, NJ 08901. The only exception to this prohibition is "fair use" as defined by U.S. copyright law.

References to internet websites (URLs) were accurate at the time of writing. Neither the author nor Rutgers University Press is responsible for URLs that may have expired or changed since the manuscript was prepared.

♾ The paper used in this publication meets the requirements of the American National Standard for Information Sciences—Permanence of Paper for Printed Library Materials, ANSI Z39.48-1992.

rutgersuniversitypress.org

Contents

Preface   vii

The Road   1

Waiting   6

Angel   19

Heartsore   34

Presents   41

Andrew   50

Diversity   62

Bethal   71

Safari   85

Goodness   93

Jokers   108

Yvonne   116

God   129

Mama Zulu   137

Security   152

Noeline   163

The Circle   176

Confessions   183

Acknowledgments 197
Notes 199
Index 215

Preface

(Skip this part for the next one if you want to start the story. If you want to know how I wrote it, keep reading.)

This is a story of a home and the people inside it, as well as those underneath.

It was built on top of a graveyard.

The buried were left behind when their families were forced to move—evicted—to make room for a new group of people. Those who live there inside the home today say they are *like* family—just not quite fully.

Life in the home bristles and burns with its own funny fervor because of the way its mixed bag of like-a-family members must get along. They either pay to live there or get paid to help the others keep on living. The little like-a-family is mostly medical professionals like nurses and caregivers (nursing assistants or aides), or they are mostly frail residents. It is a nursing, or "old age," home.

This story you are about to read is real. It is based on seven years of immersive research inside and nearby the home I call Grace, which exists somewhere in present-day South Africa. In a range of one-week- to four-month-long visits in 2015, 2017, 2019, and 2022, I spent twenty to thirty hours per week there, where I helped to feed, move, and accompany residents, joined in leisure and spiritual activities, and aided staff in nonclinical duties, observing residents' "activities of daily living" and the home's daily goings-on. Outside Grace, I visited other old age homes in the area as well as staff members' communities. I went on staff shopping and business errands and occasional daytrips for residents to church or the nearby safari park.

During this time, I met several individuals whose stories showed me—and can show all of us, perhaps—how the end of life reconditions the way we might face our past, or dimensions of it that still hauntingly linger in the present.

Here, that past is apartheid. For those who do not know or have forgotten, apartheid—meaning "separateness"—was system of racial segregation and

vii

viii PREFACE

dispossession in South Africa directed by a white-minority government against its majority black citizens and other citizens of color. Part of it involved the forced, mass removal of these peoples from their lands, as was the case for the community that formerly lived in the place that came to be known as Grace.

The white-supremacist policies and logics for apartheid had partial origins and connections to the United States of America, Great Britain, Germany, and other imperial nation-states, even as it was grounded in South Africa and affected its neighboring countries the most. It lasted for nearly fifty years, from 1948 to 1994, ending through on-the-ground protests, guerrilla warfare, and international sanctions. To lay it bare, it was violent.

The year 2024 marks thirty years since apartheid's supposed ending. What, or who still remains in its wake—an unhealed wound, a scar, a ghost—is another haunting question, as well as the question of what's yet to come. The current passing of the aging generation of apartheid's primary promoters, resisters, those in-between, and their children—some of the people you will soon meet—is a possible turning point for the future of the country and others like it that mirror its history and present-day social and racial inequalities. It is a point of reckoning.

The stories of the people of Grace and the juxtapositions that color their daily lives show that there are no easy answers to these questions. Importantly, they show how everyday conversations about racism and remembering violence are transformed in the face of aging and dying. Namely, these topics were tempered by recognition of care needs and imminent mortality, and, in turn, an understanding that we all share the same fate. In seeing this, I believe they found something like "grace" to behold these truths and go on living together, for a while longer.

The stories they shared with me more so reflect their concerns for their families, memories of the bitter and sweet moments that marked their lives, and how they juggled different identities over the course of their lives—as daughters, wives, mothers, and grandmothers, as sons and husbands, as spouses and widows, and now as caregivers and receivers. Still, the history of segregation and racial violence cannot be displaced in any version of their stories. This history undeniably shaped their respective roles in the home, varied friendships or distaste for each other, and their erasure.

By "erasure," I mean that in long-term elder care around the world, ageism, racism, and sexism push older adults and the mostly people of color who care for them to the periphery of our communities, effectively devaluing and erasing them from public life. For the staff, who are also mostly younger, working-class black women, it is a place of wage labor to make a living amid mass unemployment. For the residents, who are mostly older, middle- and working-class white women, it is a place to go on living when no one else cares for them or no one wants to. There are exceptions to these divisions, but despite and because of them, they find themselves tied together within larger systems of oppression.

In the case of Grace, however, that "funny fervor" I mentioned ignites something between people who are radically different or historically primed to be

PREFACE   ix

enemies. They find instead that they are dependent on each other—like a family, maybe.

The book you are about to read is based on field notes I wrote during and after the hours and days I spent at Grace, and, most importantly, multiple, consenting, in-depth interviews and conversations I had with staff, residents, and visitors. From all of those who I met across seven years, I chose seven to feature—three staff members, three residents, and the manager—to shine light on what reckoning with racism and much more looks like at life's end.

To hear this story, we'll take something like a daylong tour through Grace and nearby it, moving room to room or place to place to meet each of them as they go about their lives:

Seven years in a day.

To some of you, this might sound unusual. (I hope you find it enticing.)

In form then, this book is a work of creative, narrative nonfiction. It is grounded in research in a real place and time and with real people. Anthropologists like me tend to write books called ethnographies. These are also nonfiction books that feature unique individuals and explore how turns and twists in their lives are due of larger social, political, or environmental forces. They're written in the past tense and meant to make you feel as if you've come to know someone perhaps quite different than you, on their own terms.

This book does some of this but with a few creative, experimental, or wishful turns and twists—like a daydream, perhaps, wandering through time. This approach can go by different names like "literary ethnography" or "creative ethnographic nonfiction." It can also include poetry. And mystery.

I took this journey using a map set out by writer and anthropologist Kirin Narayan.[1] She outlines how a book like this one should include the following: complex, memorable characters who yearn for something that might complete them (seven in all, check); a situation where it all takes place (an endearing little old age home, check); pivotal scenes where the characters, me the writer, and you the reader interact (check); and the story itself, or the insights and personal transformations we come to experience in each encounter (check). Much of what you'll read unfolds in these pivotal scenes of character interaction—in *conversational narrative*, like a screenplay—to tell the story itself.

Because the situation of being inside a place like Grace may be unfamiliar to you, the story also requires some summaries or more background information than a conversation can behold (check). Throughout the tour, you'll come across these summaries, what legendary speculative science fiction and fantasy writer Ursula K. Le Guin called "expository lumps," or moments of *reflective narrative*. These aren't meant to be didactic—or too teacherly—but instead let you appreciate what's going on and understand why something is pivotal.

Bits of the narrative, both reflective and conversational, show up in parentheses. They're words and thoughts that made sense to me in writing this book and made the final cut. Maybe they show you what Freud and others call the superego, that part of us that wrestles with ideas and values that our parents, heroes, or communities tell us are right or wrong, and what we personally wish for instead. A perfect balance between the two is impossible, and knowing this generates conscience. These parentheses are not behind-the-scenes or diary-like filler, then, but key imports of mind, times, and relations from outside the main narrative that constellate my story of Grace—any story really—in total.[2]

Overall, *God's Waiting Room* braids together these conversational and reflective narratives, in lines of speech, thought, feeling, and memories—mine, yours, the characters—to tighten past and present into a singular rope we can use to pull ourselves toward that reckoning I mentioned.

This form of time, of a braided-together past and present, is something we all live with even if we're not often aware of it. Turning seven years into a single day is a deliberate move I make for a few reasons.

First, it is to show you the integrative experience of recollecting seven years of life to tell a single story. The process of reviewing, remembering, and writing is part of any storytelling journey, and I believe the experience of this process should somehow be honored in the end. It also foregrounds the fact that every time we (re)read a book it is a journey of rediscovery, another time to hear or learn something new about a topic and ourselves. Both are also always changing from what they once were. It puts *us*—who we are, both past and present—in the story.

Second, it is to show the experience I had of speaking with people who already braid together past and present in unexpected ways. Sometimes this is associated with short-term memory loss, dementia, or Alzheimer's disease, when people living with these conditions forget, misremember, or recollect in ways that surprise us or confound our expectations or how a story should unfold. This need not be seen as a pathological problem. Theories of gerotranscendence suggest, in part, that many older adults around the world can redefine self, space, and time in a less linear and more cosmic perspective as they age.[3] So, at some points, I pepper the story with my own and others' flashbacks and flash-forwards as flashpoint summaries to show how things ended up as life went on for some, and as it ended for others.

And third, the move to make this story into a daylong tour is to quicken our pace, and, importantly, run away from ideas that aging and dying are only yet to come, or that racism is in the past. These are active forces affecting us all and happening now, in the present. Thus, this book is written in the present tense. While this may obscure the yearslong work I put in to build trust with the people of Grace—and most people in general do not fully open up to strangers in a single day—setting this story in the past can obscure the fact that some of them are still alive today and ever-changing from who they once were. The present tense also conveys how uncertainty often marks our real, everyday encounters with others, and how we—me and these people, and maybe you—might find grace in such moments to move forward.

Again, these are real people's stories—sad, reflective, funny, curt, and sometimes shockingly nasty—that reflect complex identities and a need for ethical represen-

PREFACE xi

tation. As for aspects of some people's gender and sexual identities, I've used their own self-identifying terms. Unless drawn from direct quotes, I've mostly used "older" as the inclusive term to describe many people's identities related to age. And to represent racial aspects of some people's identities, I chose to use "black," as it is used in South Africa, rather than capitalize it as is now somewhat standard in the United States, where I live. Capitalizing "Black" can emphasize collective, historic resistance to exceptional forces of racist oppression undertaken by people of color and of African descent in both places, and yet resisting capitalization can defy further codifications or divisions that would thwart global possibilities of solidarity and freedom.[4]

These are also people who let me go forward with using their real names. Only one character, "Frikkie," is compositional, meaning someone whose scene and story I re-created based on interviews and conversations with several individuals I came to know and only to ends which creative nonfiction allows.[5] Invoking this speech from a time outside of the main narrative's time and flow, like an echo, I also use parentheses and italics for our conversation in her chapter. The manager, the woman who let this all happen by giving me permission to revisit over the years, has a real name that is not "Angel," but I've characterized her as such given that her persona meant so much more than she'd otherwise say about herself as a gatekeeper.[6]

It was also from Angel that I learned the phrase "God's waiting room" and found it compelling. It locates a sense of immensity that comes in the face of final judgments—legal, historical, human and more-than-human—and self-reflections we conjure as we meet a threshold like the one we are about to pass through.

To save the actual home from bad faith criticisms or other misreadings, I named it Grace instead of using its real name. I also chose the name to make you think about what grace is or can do to people who come into its glow.

To me, grace may be something like gentleness, a vital and possibly more-than-human force that emanates between us or from another mysterious source.[7] To me, it stands for that fervor, that bristling and burning encounter we experience with others who at first appear radically different, but through whom we come to see part of ourselves, and journey together to that future reckoning.

God's Waiting Room

The Road

On any road trip you'll need two things to make it out alive: a map, and snacks.

To make the best of both, as in how to read the map and where to get the best bites, you'll need help from locals, folks at those roadside oases who let you know you're on *their* turf, might warm to or welcome you or give you directions, bid you goodbye in your passing, and—*Jesus!*

In the rearview mirror, the grill of semi-trailer truck looks like it will be the last thing I will ever see if I don't step on the gas for this turnoff.

The rush roars by and the rented Toyota scuds to dusty stop. We—yes, you and me—are at a crossroads. I'm going to need to look at Google Maps, meaning the screenshots I took from it this morning at the Airbnb where I had Wi-Fi. There's no reception out here. For me at least.

At the crossroads, a rusting sign arrows left to Nelspruit, the letters of the name faded by sunlight and time. Another sign points in the same direction, in new reflective lettering, to Mbombela—two names for the same place.

This is where one of the road trip necessities comes in handy—a map.

Maps are what made me want to learn more about South Africa and travel here in the first place. At that time, it was ten years after an old way of life here ended— "apartheid," more on that soon—and a new one emerged. Our local ten-page newspaper even wrote a story about my trip. It felt *that* extraordinary to the folks in my small town.

That small-town life in the American Midwest was not *so*, so uniform as you'd think. Among the Indigenous and immigrant people in the area—Polish, Hmong, German, Oneida, Irish, Menominee—there are lots of Belgians and Dutch. A look at the phone book in days past or the stands of the football games we went to on Friday nights (American football, not soccer) showed a lot of Van Enkenvoorts, Van Laanens, Vander Bergs, Vanden Bergs, Vanden Langen Bergs, and the like.

On older maps of this country, you see a lot of similar-looking names— Langebaan, Berg, Vanderbijlpark, Vereeniging, voortrekker things, Van der this and Van der that.

I knew enough then somehow, and learned more later, as to why it wasn't by chance that there are people like this—and by that I mean white people in general—all over the world today.

(Settler colonial bullshit.)

I believe "old ways of life" or "old ways of thinking" we often talk about are like ghosts. They don't die off completely and get supplanted when "new" ways come about. The "new" is usually a reformulation of what came before, or a resurrection of something that laid dormant and reappears in different form and is heard for the first time by a new generation. The writer Jarred Thompson reminded me that ghosts are stuck in time loops. They repeat past stories when they reappear and usually flashback to the traumatic. Like ghosts, we might not notice the "old ways" among us at first, but they're always still with us—never entirely absent or forgettable.

We stand where we do today because of the choices made by those who came before us, or the choices some were forced by others to make. We've inherited a still unequal, but ever-changing world that was created, in part, by past generations, whose ghosts are also somehow still here: in their descendants who walk among us as strangers or soon-to-be-friends—some locals we'll soon meet, maybe—and in the very words we have to describe the world and where exactly it is we're standing or going. Like a city with two names.

This all may be too obvious, and yet I still believe in ghosts.

Looking up from the phone, I see what else we needed for the road trip—snacks, netted bags full of them hanging as yummy drapery from the awning of a market stall, a forest of feathery blue gumtrees framing the scene behind it. There are some truly subtropical options here in the "land of the rising sun"—Mpumalanga, the lowveld region of South Africa—oranges from groves hueing the horizon, softball-sized avocados (not the bumpy Haas kind that go on pricy toast), and nuts.

Groundnuts (sort of like peanuts) are Indigenous and richly cluster beneath many black families' farms around here. Macadamias are newer. They're mostly grown in white-owned agro-industrial orchards whose owners came to take up most of the arable land here over several decades and leave a big water footprint in the age of a drying climate. Since 2020, the lowveld's been the world's biggest producer of macadamias. They're expensive. And they don't usually sell the two kinds in a mixed bag.

No one's around at the stall yet.

We'll wait.

The car's clammy conditioned air blows over my fingers as I flick away the screenshot map and open Instagram. First is a selfie. With a sexy smirk, my friend wears a T-shirt that says, "F-ck your Racist Grandma." It gets dozens of heart reactions. I know it's meant for me—for white people generally—to think about.

THE ROAD

Googling where to buy it—Splendid Rain Co.—and reading more, I learn that for the creator, Olatiwa Karade, the phrase is personal. She was once in a relationship with a partner whose mother told her, "I don't feel comfortable with you being in my family if I can't touch your hair." The mother said that "because they were first generation immigrants, they didn't know any other word for Black people other than Negroes, so to excuse her behavior because she just doesn't know any better." Karade felt that her partner's mother was "just excusing [her] own bigotry," and for Karade, merchandizing this slogan could "normalize pro-Blackness by making it attractive and accessible." You can get the phrase printed on tote bags and COVID face masks.[1]

Suddenly, from the woods, an older woman appears.

Before I crank the parking brake, she's back at the stall, wearing a black and white NASCAR windbreaker, a wrap skirt, and a black fuzzy beret. From her waist, like a belt, a thin, dried grass rope—the last is a bit of "traditional" garb. It means she's been widowed or mourning for her son or brother. Men tend to die sooner than women everywhere in the world, and some men sooner than others, from seemingly "natural," "accidental," or "senseless" things that are in fact systemically violent and racial.[2]

People who look like me here tend to get the "special price, my friend" introduction to market stall goods like nuts, but today, I'm someone else.

"*Mntanam*'" (My child), she says, eyes glimmering like the residual impression of lightning—cataracts, maybe, or something celestial.

And I to her: "*Yebo, mama*" (I see you, mama).

I don't think we're starting off on quite the right terms—me in my late thirties, somewhere in between the Gen Xers and Millennials, she in her early sixties. She's a mother to someone, for sure, if not her own, then a sister's children, or honorably to other people's children and the men around the neighborhood. To me, she looks "older" than a mama.

I think that if we want to go by the age-as-a-thing-of-honor equation, I should've called her *gogo* instead ("grandmother," a more respectful term for older women here). And she, to me, *baba* ("father," the appropriate one for a man my age, I think).

Here though, for someone who looks like me, "baba" also means "sir."

Sometimes, miscommunication happens because of that mess of words and languages we've inherited from the past, where we talk to but past each other because we've failed to mutually understand or share the meanings and impacts of what we communicate to each other.

Sometimes, this happens because we have wrong ideas about other people and vice versa. Usually, because of the "old ways" or forces that are bigger than any one of us, others may come to believe you're reducible to a single dimension. Or that you're unchanging in their mind's eye, aspects of your character fixed forever as they knew you at one point in time. As the world moves on or changes, they go with it. You do not. You become a reference point for them to define themselves: a stereotype.

Be it surrounding your race, who you sleep with or are attracted to, or how old you are, it is an idea about you that haunts you wherever you go.

Reckoning with these ideas others put upon us can mean reclaiming them, changing them into signs of pride among those who are like us and the like-minded as an act of self-certitude. To me, it must also mean sharing more—a testimony or confession, maybe—as to who we are, where we've been, and where we hope to go, with those like-minded people as well as others who at first may seem too radically different to fathom. Talking to, and not past each other, beyond false or haunting ideas we have of each other. I believe this can generate means to envision and create a better world than the one we've inherited, or at least an alternative place in the meantime—an "Elsewhere."

Black, Indigenous, and other scholars, activists, and artists of color anoint this Elsewhere we may dream of creating an "Otherwise" world.[3] To make it there also entails a road trip of sorts, a "walk" in Nelson Mandela's words,[4] or rather clearing out and making our own path alongside or counter to those we already have on the map. It entails uncomfortable conversation, critical reflection, and strategic action so that we can counteract what the hands of history have dealt to us. These are means to get to a postpostcolonial, no-bullshit place—to freedom. It will take time.

And come to think of it, those racist grandmas and grandpas might be almost out of it. They're about to become the next generation of ghosts. And again, even as they depart from this world, they're going to remain with us in some form or another.

We might want to do something in the meantime, before they go, to encourage them to change their tune—to prevent or free them perhaps, from haunting us later.

To me, that will mean first accepting the fact of their ongoing presence once their mortal coil finishes its burn—that racism is not going to be over anytime soon or in the near future, whether we like it or not. (We should not, obviously.) And practically, I believe that will mean taking time to talk with members of older generations, racist or not, before they're gone—to hear what their motives were in making part of this world we've inherited and what *they* hope comes next for it. In doing so—if we go by the age-as-honorable equation—we can honor both who they were and are now.

We may find that these older adults have already changed their tune, meaning they already have complex or changed ideas about the world and others in it, sharing perspectives—or a testimony or confession, perhaps—that empower us to transform parts of this world we find intolerable. And we may also be transformed in the process of hearing these, in ways that show us that we often traffic in ageist assumptions about others. Facing the end of one's proverbial road—one's life itself—usually put things in an altogether different light.

A few crumpled bills pass from my sweaty hand to her callused one to get a netted bag full of nuts and oranges that's enough for ten kids' school lunches. She'd call

THE ROAD 5

this *umphako*, or food you take on a journey. My family, my person—Mom and Dad, Charlie—are back home. I'm on this one alone for now.

Back in the car, I wonder, "How do you do all this, mama?" or gogo, rather—rise, travel, vend, wait.

A powerline pole nearby the stall is papered with ads—a pancake and golf fundraiser for an old age home, Herbalife, auto mechanics, Dr. Swami's magic charms for a bigger penis, love, and fortune, Pastor and Lady Pastor Smuts's all-night service for divine grace at the union hall.

Above us, the powerlines singe-crackle in a coronal language. It sounds as if somebody's calling from another side of the sky.

At the crossroads, which way will you to go to make it to Heaven, I wonder. What signs will you see, and how will you read them? Who will you meet?

At this highway crossroads, you can go left to Nelspruit/Mbombela as the two signs said, or right to the airport called Kruger. It lands you near one of the biggest safari parks on the continent. Getting directions, gogo tells me she lives at home with her granddaughters at Dwaleni—"the Rock"—a township behind the airport's fences. It's where her parents were forcibly relocated to a generation ago from where they lived in a nearby small town we're headed to next. Some never made the move to the Rock:

The buried ones who were left behind.

Back to the map. However large or small in scale, a view from that Elsewhere or Otherwise can also show that "home" might never just be a single, physical place. Home can be a state of mind, a perpetual state of creating bonds with other people—those who are like-minded or like-a-family, those who are radically different, or even ghosts—and the work of mutually minding those bonds. Home might be a matter of *whom* rather than *where*, a matter of making good or right with others, of making a good life, and living out that life wherever that may be.

And back to the map, one last time. Be it a condo or flat, McMansion, or an old age home, you can't deny that home will also be a physical place. One hopes that it will be a place to thrive, rest, and evoke a sense of respite and freedom. We hope it will be a kind of dream house for the time being, for our time remaining in this world. That its greenspace, walls, rooms, and us—as caretakers, caregivers, or both—order what we hope will feel like the opposite of captivity.

Still though, I wonder, *who* will be home?

Listen.

Someone is knocking.

Waiting

"Ooo, a sexy man."

In an instant, like we're drinking up each other's gaze at a bar, the words spoken from her magenta lips prick my ear.

It's not the first thing I thought I'd hear from an angel, as I somehow believe she could be, or among the clinking, shuffling, and other 8:00 A.M. noises of a nursing home—"old age home" as they're called here. No bar then, either, of course, but I do smell cigarette smoke.

Recombobulating a lanyard thick with keys, a thermos and accordion folder, and her half-zipped fleece—the morning shift juggle—she lets me know she's got more coming for me, adding, "just wait here a minute, sweetie."

From the sign on the door she rushes into, I see she's actually the manager. Her office opens onto the waiting room, which is where we're standing now, bathed in the warm light of the sun shining down through the yellow fiberglass roof. Beside the print of Van Gogh's golden field of sunflowers is another bright standout, a brass plaque in Afrikaans commemorating the home's founding in the 1950s, as well as a certificate in English showing they passed their monthly health inspection. Next to that, a sign with the home's name:

"Grace,"

And their mission statement: "To render 24-hour quality comprehensive nursing care to needy frail aged and disabled persons of all racial groups."

Just a few of the things to read while we size up the place.

They used to give you lots more to read in waiting rooms like this. Magazines like *Essence, Drum, Newsweek, Sports Illustrated.* Nowadays, the physical copies and subscriptions are pretty much all canceled. They assume you brought your phone to keep yourself busy. Canceling subscriptions save them a few bucks each month but also waste their time. For us—visitors and patients—our phones open a Pandora's box of questions to ask our providers, culled from browser searches, WebMD, and family group chats with your aunties' latest medical findings from

Facebook. Now we're armed with self-diagnoses, average-starred ratings for the place, and last-minute guesses as to what will happen to us next.

A waiting room is what we might call a liminal zone, an unusual place betwixt and between worlds where you make new or unexpected relationships with the folks you find in there with you. Some easy examples are the lifelong bonds borne among those who make a sort of transition together, like military boot campers, pledging sorority sisters, or some teenage boys in this country who undergo ritual circumcision during school vacation as part of becoming men.[1]

Another might be a group of souls who find themselves trapped together somewhere—an elevator stuck between two floors, a desert island, a prison, or maybe someplace like this. Make do with each other in order to survive.

Another might be purgatory. Make do with yourself, because it might feel like an insufferable forever until you make up for what you've done wrong to get out of there.

In the meantime, this bright cell feels comfortable enough. Cute too—beside a couch, a few teddy bears smile from the top of a pile of knitted potholders and beanie hats with heart-shaped price tags—a soft confinement between the "real world" we entered from the parking lot—outside, wild, free—and the world of the home—inside, masked, secure.

Somewhere behind the brick wall, something guttural is growling:

Someone's sleep apnea, I guess.

Just be patient, sweetie.

Wait.

Let's go back to how we got here in the first place, again by way of a road trip.

The early 2010s—in the United States, we were into the first few years of Obamacare, the snarky Republican rebrand of the Democrat-championed Patient Protection and Affordable Care Act and its riders like the Elder Justice Act. The Affordable Care Act aimed to expand health insurance protections and coverage to the vast majority American citizens, including the most vulnerable, who'd never be able to pay out of pocket for catastrophically expensive medical care. It drove more of us, especially then-underinsured black and Hispanic peoples, into the insurance market on both public and private plans.[2]

All Republican members of Congress, and all white at that time as far as I can tell, voted against it. They took to radio and TV airwaves and small-town diners to frame it as lethal. Of the many attempts to repeal it, the first bill was titled "Repealing the Job-Killing Health Care Law Act." They said there'd be "death panels," which many older adults still believe in.[3] Successively, they chopped away many of the act's components, and the Elder Justice Act was stalled for a decade.[4] Really, it came at the greatest expense to the health and welfare of Republicans' own constituents.[5] Under pretense that it was an economic affront to freedom, they really did it to smear the Affordable Care Act's main promoter—the first black president.

Around the same time, South Africa was also making inroads to support its most vulnerable citizens by drafting the National Health Insurance (NHI) plan. NHI is a plan to liberate the health care system from its sordid past and bifurcated present. Here, if you become sick, injured, or disabled, your options are to go to either a public or private facility. By and large, the country's black majority use "free" public facilities because for decades they were systematically denied more substantive health care and means to pay for it. Better-equipped facilities are private where you pay out of pocket or use a medical aid scheme, an insurance-type policy you subscribe to or get through your employer. Even for the those who can afford medical aid—they're a minority of South Africans and mostly white—it often gets used up late in the year, forcing you back into public facilities or out-of-pocket payments.

Today's divisions are the historical outcome of white South Africans' segregation and dispossession of people of color, which expanded over hundreds of years through wars and colonization, and more recently, nearly fifty years of racist government policies known as apartheid, which only formally ended in 1994—again, more on that soon.

The NHI plan is meant to rectify those past wrongs. It aims to build more nursing schools and improve public facilities, labs, and IT. It proposes more community health programs and public health messaging about personal preventive care—add less salt to the stew and less sugar to your tea, please. It has a national tax with pro-business aspects like a progressive rate structure. It tries to coax providers back into public facilities—many doctors fled the public sector in the last years of apartheid.[6] All of this will hopefully diminish the racial inequalities built into health care and raise life expectancy to a ripe older age of seventy for all men and women by 2030. In 2016, it was a less ripe sixty-seven for non-blacks and an even less ripe fifty-seven for black people.[7] Since COVID, it's dropped further.[8]

So, to compare what happened in the United States to here and what it all meant for older people and people who work in health care, like an anthropologist might do, I went on a road trip—to Mpumalanga, the land of the rising sun—to where they tried to roll it out.

At first, I met dozens of health care workers and medical aid brokers in their halogen-lit hospital, clinic, and mini-mall offices, or, a favorite spot for some, Wimpy's restaurant—picture vinyl booths festooned with kids' birthday party balloons and milkshake splatters on the walls.

Most of the people I met and spoke to were white. They said NHI would never happen, was a dream, or "a pie in the sky" in one doctor's words. They believed public and private could not come together, and they feared going to the former which was also too broken to fix. Many had experienced bad care in public facilities or did not want the same to happen to their families. Nothing they saw in NHI would make a substantial improvement in anyone's lives, let alone for older adults, they believed. Everyone would need to be on board—nobody was—and it would take a lifetime to work.

I learned that medical aid schemes that some of the brokers sold did not even help their own aging parents. Long-term care costs—like paying for an old age

WAITING 9

homestay—were excluded. Most told their customers not to add parents to policies because their premiums would skyrocket. Again, it's mostly middle- to upper-class white families who have medical aid, unless you're a government employee, for which you have GEMS (Government Employees Medical Scheme). The acronym eerily reflects the hoards of diamonds excavated for companies like DeBeers by generations of black miners here. Today, many of these men, now retired, make massive aid claims to cover treatment costs for silicosis and tuberculosis they contracted on the job.

Health care workers and brokers' answers to my questions about costs and possibilities for more equitable care drew out something similar to what happened around Obamacare. In both places, attempts to build better systems and spaces to care for people—including elder care, something we may all inevitably need in some form as part of being human—were stymied by white anxieties.

Leveling the playing field felt impossible for these white people I spoke to, perhaps because it presented a debilitating albeit unreal prospect. To them, changing care access somehow meant they would get *less* as others got *more*, be it treatment, financial support, or continuous care. In a way, in South Africa and the United States, two countries historically shaped by white supremacy, changing the system for older people in particular, or all people in general, would erase the privileged differences that long defined a part of who they were—it would somehow make white people feel "less than." In a way, it would make them feel black.[9]

Despite these concerns and just two weeks prior to the May 2024 national elections, marking thirty years since the 1994 vote that ended white-minority rule, President Cyril Ramaphosa signed the NHI bill into law.

To me, there had to be more to this story: about how racism affected older adults—the way it shapes how they see themselves and others, conditions their access to care and who becomes their caregivers—about how considering racism could help us make sense of ageism, and more.[10]

Amid the Wimpy's milkshake splatters, one broker I met suggested I visit an old age home to see how people were cared for in practice rather than policies like the NHI.

I found this one—Grace—on Google Maps, just off the main road.

~

The driveway to Grace meets a remote-controlled sliding gate and electrified fence. A woman with a name tag that says Pretty sits in a small house. She's private security. Most places in this country with said-to-be valuable, rare, or fragile people, animals, or things inside have it.

"Who do you want to see here?" Pretty commands.

"The manager, please. For a tour," I chirp. (Or to see if there's an open spot for gogo or grandpa—another normal visit here, I bet.) She pens our details on her clipboard.

First impressions: great landscaping. Scarlet poinsettias, sago palms, and crown of thorns bushes flourish among perfect little rows of what I guess are one-bed, one-bath brick cottages. The clean uniformity looks like the planned neighborhood Mom and Dad downsized to a few years ago, leaving a two-story McMansion-looking house—it was the 1990s—with a yard I hated mowing as a kid. Their new single-story home's a good fit for them, like their mostly older adult neighbors in general—no stairs for creaky knees, less space to keep up, contractors who mow the lawn and shovel snow. They know their neighbors in this little village. In gerontological terms, they can age in place.

And what about the people here?

We'll see.

The drive up from the gate to the main house passes a scrubby grass field that appears to be empty, except for a few small, sun-bleached wooden stakes that mark out a sort of zone.

(They look like grave markers, I think.)

Maybe it marks something underneath that's dangerous like a gas line, or vital like water.

Maybe it's keeping something down that's been waiting to get out.

~

Homes like Grace are not your typical senior housing option in this country. By comparison, in the United States there are nearly fifty thousand long-term care facilities, with more than two million residents—the majority are white.[11] By 2030, all members of the baby boomer generation, born just after World War II, will be sixty-five years of age or older and facing attendant, often long-term care needs of this new chapter of life. In South Africa there are little more than a thousand such homes where fewer than 4 percent of residents are black.[12]

Old age homes here were first set up around the turn of the twentieth century by and for whites. In the 1920s, the government commissioned the American Carnegie Corporation to study poorer whites—mostly Afrikaner farmers and foresters at the time as whites of British descent commandeered mining and other industries—with aims to improve their lot and help differentiate them from the needs and lives of the black majority.[13] Soothing the plight of poorer older whites became a major social welfare policy and was promoted with nationalist flair as the prerogative of white women to uplift families of the white nation with motherly zeal.[14] The government established a state pension for white older adults first, and charities built more whites-only old age homes.[15]

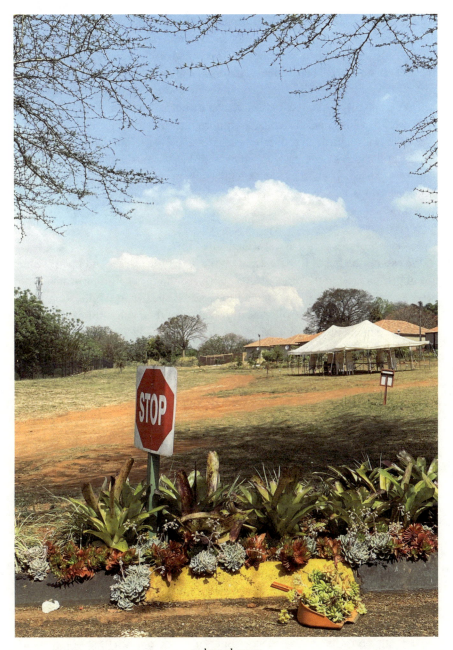

a cleared space

By the end of the 1940s, the whites-only National Party began to implement policies around a principle of apartheid, meaning to "separate" "race groups" in all practical means of life: no interracial marriage or sex, no nonwhite ownership of land, racially separate schools and public spaces, and, eventually, altogether separate territories. In the 1950s and 1960s, the white government expanded its "native reserves" policies for black peoples and expelled many thousands more from urban and suburban neighborhoods to rural reservations they then called "homelands" according to what they believed to be black people's correct "tribes." They set up puppetized black administrators and allocated a pitiful amount of support for development.[16] This included money for those administrators' salaries, as well as blacks-only schools, clinics, and, interestingly, plans for old age homes.[17]

Slowly, the white model for collectively housing unrelated older adults got off the ground in black homeland communities. Later, a few black individuals and organizations built homes on their own, some with help from the diaspora as part of global anti-apartheid efforts.[18] Soon after the unbanning of black political parties in the 1990s, admissions to schools, clinics, and places like Grace became race-blind. Apartheid "ended," and everyone could now live where they pleased. Supposedly.

The residents of this Grace lived through all of this.

We can do the math. If the normal intake is sixty-five years and up for senior housing, then most of the residents were born around the beginning of apartheid, between the 1930s and 1950s. As young and middle-aged white adults, some probably resisted or spoke out against the degradation of their fellow human beings of color. Some likely promoted it. Many just lived with it—being untouched or not the target of racist ire—so as to raise families, enjoy weekends, and grow older as if it were all so normal. To many, it was. Some even say they were truly oblivious to all of it until the 1970s. In the 1990s, in middle age, they faced the world-changing transition of people of color gaining their freedom.

Today, in late life, they're waiting for another change, in soon moving from this life to the next. We'll see what they're doing in the meantime.

~

I'm not getting impatient for the angel, but the aroma lingering into the waiting room revs another guttural sound inside me: stomach growlings. The table-top crumbs and empty teacups I see in the nearby dining room complete the end-of-breakfast scene. (It was probably a mistake to only have coffee at the Airbnb this morning and a handful of the nuts I bought from gogo.)

All the diners have left except for one, a white woman in a heart-appliquéd sweater. She's scowling at us—maybe angry or shocked, I can't tell—or at something past us that's invisible.

Checking my phone to see how long we've been in here, means seeing I haven't closed Instagram yet: my friend's selfie with the T-shirt call to get rid of racist grandma shines brightly on the screen.

It's an age-specific version of what South Africans may know from the recent years' news: the infamous "F-CKWHITEPEOPLE" print created by genderqueer artist and activist Dean Hutton. For their Master of Art project, Hutton printed the phrase on a wall, chair, and pair of boots for a show in the South African National Museum. After that, a white nationalist group, the Cape Party, sued the Museum in the Equality Court for promoting hate speech in staging Hutton's art. The court found the museum did not promote it.

In the view of Judge Daniel Mafeleu Thulare, the big-lettered phrase "properly contextualized and understood" meant "to reject, confront and dismantle structures, systems, knowledge, skills and attitudes of power that keep white people racist." In the full ruling, the judge used other language that seemed to dispel phantoms similar to racist grandmas. According to Thulare, Hutton aimed to create a "change of mindset, a paradigm shift from the old ways," "old practice and ancient formulae" in order to "keep pace with the requirements of changing conditions in South Africa."[19]

So, out with the old, in with the new?

Psychologists like to ask whether older adults are more racist in general or if they're dysregulated and more impressionable.[20] Sociologists and media studies scholars argue for the United States at least that the current landscape of older adults' conservative, sometimes-racist views reflects the Fox News-ification of white suburban and rural middle- and working-class people's minds.[21]

Others argue that our ideas about older people being more racist actually reflect our own ageism—prejudiced beliefs that older people are problematic by being from another era or have views of the world that went unchanged for the second half of a lifetime.[22]

If someone is both older and racially problematic to illegal extremes, there is no age limit for their prosecution and incarceration, either. Some countries easily sentence old racists to prison, like former Nazis in Germany—Josef Schütz was 101 in 2022 when he was sentenced to five years in prison for being an accessory to the murder of 3,518 people at Sachsenhausen concentration camp during World War II. In the United States, legal technicalities may flout this push, like the grand jury decision to not indict eighty-eight-year-old Carolyn Bryant Donham for kidnapping and manslaughter, also in 2022. Known internationally, Donham was a white American woman whose false accusation that Emmet Till harassed her led her husband and his half-brother to lynch Till, a fourteen-year-old black boy, in 1955.

Before the grand jury commenced, images surfaced of Donham on the porch of her Kentucky home receiving hospice care for cancer, a nasal cannula strung from her jowls.

For a lot of observers on X (formerly Twitter) then, age and frailty didn't matter—they'd find a way to get her. Prison, or something more physical, was the justice she deserved.[23]

Donham died a year later.

White people tend to live longer compared to people of color in most multiracial countries.[24] I believe it is the outcome of white supremacy, or "white sovereignty," as some call it, an outcome of violence against people of color—outright in killings and or structural mutations that lead to unequal health care systems, discrimination in policing, segregation, and maldistribution of life-supporting services and resources. Like food, or health insurance.

Today, some white people's aging and dying seems to signal a historical turning point of the "old ways" of thinking and doing things I mentioned. Like colonialism. Many people of color in postcolonial countries the world over celebrated the deaths of Queen Elizabeth II and Prince Philip, for example. Or at least they chose not to mourn.[25]

The idea of a supposed turning point of this kind also makes many white people anxious or nervous.[26] In the United States, psychiatrist and sociologist Jonathan Metzl shows worsening health outcomes and mortality rates for poorer white people twin to an *imagined* population-demographic shift where black people and people of color will eventually outnumber white people. This imagined shift or change for that country also converges with the reality that its mostly white baby boomer generation—many of them children of the hero-ized "greatest generation"—continues to age further into late life. Today, fears that white people and their power will be diminished are at the fore in conspiratorial "replacement theories" and ideas of "white genocide" that incite some white nationalists to political culture wars, protests, and mass shootings in places like grocery stores.[27] These same conspiracies exist and resurface in places where whites have always been a racial minority but have long held economic and political power, like South Africa.

I wonder whether older white people's dying means an end to systems of white supremacy that they created, were complicit with, or perpetuated, or if it can mean a new era of black empowerment.

I wonder what this means for forgiveness or racial reconciliation, or change.

I wonder if older black and white people are roommates in here.

~

It doesn't matter who you are—in South Africa or anywhere—you have to wait.

Dream, wonder—maybe anxiously—when it will be your turn or what comes next.

Read the room, a magazine, or a book in the meantime.

In the 1980s, near the height of the civil and guerrilla war to end apartheid, the American anthropologist Vincent Crapanzano went to live in a little village near Cape Town. There, he met ordinary white people: middle-age, middle-class, Christian civil servants, housewives, and farmers. He wrote a book about their reflections on the past and present and titled it *Waiting*. To him, their lives evinced a peculiar, paralytic sense of time. They weren't filled with guilt or dread for the anticipated changes their country faced. Rather, they were marked by total

WAITING

banality. In other words, they made themselves boring in sitting by while South Africa was dragged to freedom. "Therein lies its pity—and its humanity," Crapanzano wrote, saying the villagers' sense of the world was "without élan, vitality, creative force. It is numb, muted, dead."[28]

But the villagers went on living. They worked, puttered, gossiped. Many passed the time going to church, which Crapanzano saw as a reaching for a spiritual something (a nothing) that would not save them from their wrong-sided place in history. Today, some of them are no longer with us, but some may still be alive—maybe in places like Grace.

In his *New York Times* review of *Waiting*, J. M. Coetzee, a South African winner of the Nobel Prize in Literature, concluded that we could somehow "sympathize" with these villagers and Crapanzano's "desire to reproduce their fullness of social experience in all its contradictions."[29] But being the son of a white middle-class South African civil servant himself, Coetzee did not believe the villagers represented the people he knew.

(For some people, a true story about their own world is hard to read. I expect it'll be the same thing here, for people whose lives are messy and don't fit our preconceived notions of who they are or ought to be.)

And still, fiction comes to mimic real life. A few years later, Coetzee wrote a book called *Age of Iron* depicting the final months of the life of one Mrs. Curren, a white elderly professor of classics—dead white people languages. Her shopping trips and doctors' visits, her searching for a relationship with her estranged daughter who left for the United States as many whites did then in fear of black retribution, her searching to understand the violence that separated her suburb from the township where her black domestic worker Florence lived—these all shorten as she dies of cancer.

As she's further absorbed in pain, absorbed into her upstairs bedroom, Mrs. Curren is cared for by Mr. Vercueil, an enigmatic black man and street dweller with whom she grows weirdly closer. In the final scene, he slips into her deathbed at her invitation.

"There is no need to feel sorry for me," she says to no one.[30]

More recent is Craig Higginson's novel *The Dream House*. It centers on an elderly white couple—wheelchair-using Patricia and her husband Richard, who lives with Alzheimer's. They wait on a dark and stormy night to vacate their haunted farmstead to downsize to an apartment on the coast. Beauty, their black domestic worker, will move with and care for them. In the twilight, they're confronted by Looksmart, their black former foster child, now a successful businessman whom they've trespassed against. The twist is that he buys their beloved farm to turn into a luxury housing development.

The Dream House touched many. An earlier play version was staged in London's West End with Academy Award nominee Janet Suzman as Patricia. The novel was used in elite South African high school graduation exams for students to think and write about important topics like their own grandparents' ways of doing things—racism and other things.

In the preface, Higginson says the couple is based on eccentric neighbors he knew as a child: a seemingly rapacious and incoherent man and his wife with "frizzy greying hair, yellow teeth like bits of sweetcorn and laughing half-hidden eyes."[31] The two sound a bit nonhuman—something older adults often get stereotyped to be.[32] Later on, he endows them with bits of humanity, saying they would be "faintly horrified by what I've made of them. . . . They were people of their time, increasingly uneasy in a world that was rapidly outstripping them."[33] Higginson later found their graves in a church cemetery.

Per the book's copyright page though, we are told *The Dream House* "is a work of fiction. Any resemblance to actual places or persons, living or dead, is purely coincidental."

(Unlike this one you're reading.)

The last and more recent book recommendation I'd give to you is one that's written by a black woman novelist: *The Woman Next Door* by Yewande Omotoso.[34] Instead of a black domestic worker and old white employer, the two main characters are peers, wealthy widows Hortensia (black) and Marion (white) in an elite Cape Town subdivision, their McMansions separated by a hedge. The two have a bemused disdain for each other, especially Hortensia for Marion's obliviousness. There's a fall—an all-too-common and debilitating injury for older adults—and they come to inhabit the same house for a while.

Waiting for her to get better, Hortensia's enemy becomes her helper. Marion's not "the help," per se, but she tries. Hortensia appreciates it, you're made to think.

I hope you like or look for some of these recommendations. (They're all on Amazon.) These and other books sort of primed my expectations as to who or what we might find in a place like Grace because there isn't much else written about old age homes today in this country.[35] That is, until COVID showed us again how people in congregate living facilities like old age homes or prisons, are multiply vulnerable, and that these can be sites of displacement—people placed out of public sight and mind.

Aside from *The Woman Next Door*, these books read a bit like familiar storylines from the United States, of black domestic workers taking care of white people—*The Help*, again, *Wit*, *Driving Miss Daisy*, or any other where underdog-yet-heroic black people work for an ungrateful older white employer who usually grows wiser to the futility of their prejudice and the humanity of people of "a different race."

Even if they are set in blockbuster films and fiction books, these roles are not so far removed from reality. In the United States at least, it is black people, people of color, recent immigrants, and mostly women who work in elder care, or in low-paid, undervalued jobs like certified nursing assistants, nurse's aides, or the like.[36]

Back home, Charlie tells me that in the ER where he works, most of the sitters—the low-paid job of watching the sick languish in their beds—are mostly Haitian women. Brazilian and Portuguese immigrant and working-class white women

WAITING 17

were the caregivers of the small-town nursing home where he first started back in the day as a nurse in training.

I wonder though if there are black nurses here who care for black residents.

I wonder what each of them think about the other,

And what they think of this place.

~

However it's differentially conditioned by white supremacy, aging is also universal. Whoever we are, we inevitably become frailer. If we make it far enough in life, aging to frailty and dying can show us powerlessness, for example, in the inability of the body, rather than our will, to hold itself together with physical integrity. Some parts come apart, and some work better than others.

Aging also shows us that however strongly we feel about our race, gender, or sexuality, these are also fleeting, sometimes-stereotypical ideas hung onto our bodies by culture. We are usually powerless to preserve these aspects of our identities as unchanging facets of ourselves. We may begin to dis-identify, or no longer see ourselves in the world itself as we once did.

Feeling virile or beautiful, for instance, is tied to sexuality and gender. These feelings can fragment as older adults may find that others are revolted by or laugh at the thought that older adults feel sexual desire or desirable. Older women especially are told they should "age gracefully," a criticism that comes with a whole set of limiting ideas about what gracefulness is or what women of a "certain age" should do or look like. (Ask Madonna about it.)

Feeling like "race doesn't matter" to one's identity, for instance, is tied to racism. People who believe that it's irrelevant if one is "white, black, yellow, or purple" are usually white themselves and would not want to live as anything but. And to others, white people in general may become stereotyped as "old racists" when they age, from entitled "Karen" types in middle age to the get-off-my-lawn and get-out-of-my-country types in older age, those of a "different time" or generation lost in the present day.

Feeling like a good mother, father, or parent, for instance, is also tied to our wishes and physical abilities to care for others. These abilities also fall away in late life. Others must now do that work, to care for you as you grow older.

You, who will wait to see what tomorrow brings.

Who will you choose to be in the passing time:

The next day, the next hour,

Next.

~

"Ooo, *goeie more!*" (good morning!)

Lost in reading the signs, the stares of teddy bears, the sudden burst of what sounds like "hooey mora" to my ears makes me jump.

"English?" I shrug, looking at her blankly—the secretary, with thin, wispy hair that flies up from the back of her neck.

She's surprised too, probably wondering, "Shouldn't you know what I'm saying?" (Or however she'd say it in Afrikaans.)

Time's up.

The little white woman wafts us the through the door,

Free from the bright cell to meet the angel.

Angel

The first thing you see is yourself, or someone who looks like your ghost.

Two flat-screen monitors midway up the wall broadcast four security camera feeds. The first feed is for the waiting room, where we came from, and the next for the room we're in now. There I am, on camera, hunched over with this old leather backpack. It looks like I need a haircut.

The other two feeds pan down a long hall, lined with doors on either side, which continually brightens out until there's nothingness at the end.

Must be a glitch. Even if it's hi-res, it's all grayscale—everyone here comes off as black and white in the camera frame at least.

Her office throne is an L-shaped desk and swivel chair with a lower-back support pad. The desk itself looks set up like a civilization-building boardgame. Mini Towers of Babel, stacks of three-ring binders of intake materials are built across the desktop—social workers' and doctors' evaluations, medical aid and funeral policies, next-of-kin contacts. They convey the legal-technical specs of the end-of-life story for each soul who lives here.

She knows more than what these docs could tell us about each one, though. In her role, she's more than just a bestuurder (manager) as her nearby business cards indicate. This job entails becoming a guardian of sorts. The mostly women like her who work in social welfare and health care help to shepherd older adults from this world to the next when they know the time is right,

Aiding elders who may soon become ancestors.

She's like an angel in a way. In my mind, that's the name she deserves.

I say *may* become ancestors, because, for now, I believe you don't automatically turn into one once you die. Both you and people like her need to make sure things are done correctly on your way out. That takes work:

Paperwork, of course, that's her specialty.

Social work, meaning that long-term care must be organized for older adults to receive it and others to give it, and that some kind of positive relationship must develop between the two for it to be successful. As older adults or frail people, we'd actually be lucky—no, privileged—to be part of this relationship. Instead, we'd die lonesome or alone. She knows each and every individual who lives and works together here. She's met and vetted them all.

And lastly, *spiritual work*, which I believe is twinned to the social part. I believe that being a good person or generating ideas about how we ought to be good to each other—what we may call morality—equips us with a kind of power. If we don't do the work to develop good long-term care relationships, for example, or if we fail to prevent aging and dying people from leaving this world on bad terms—sad, lonesome, angry, disillusioned, confused about what or who they're leaving behind and what's next—there will be spiritual consequences.

I don't believe the borders between this world and the next are so, so strong like the electrified fence outside. The borders are much more thin, almost transparent, like aged skin. I believe the dead are always around us, in the stuff they leave behind, memories of them physically revived in a scent, song, or subtle gesture made toward you by another—a glance, a kiss—and in other unexpected ways.

If we don't make good with aging and dying people, they won't see a reason to be good to us either, after they're gone. They won't become ancestors—those beings who tenderly visit us or bless us with fertility and fortune. They'll haunt us instead.

She has all the paperwork and social and spiritual skill sets on her résumé, I bet.

Behind thin gold frames, her eyes twinkle, like I imagine they would on white-bearded St. Peter or God or Santa Claus when you finally meet face-to-face after waiting bewildered in the queue. She's touched up her magenta lips in the mean-time, settling in for the interview. Her lavender French tips pinch off a few brown-ing nasturtium petals from a nearby bouquet ribboned with a notecard.

"Marie's too frail to get out for her granddaughter's wedding," she says. "Poor tannie"—meaning "auntie," more respectful, I guess, than *ouma* (grandma), or gogo—"but they brought her these yesterday. Sweet, neh?"

"Neh?" means "yeah?" as in "Yeah, don't you agree?"

"I do, neh."

"And you're a doctor?" she asks.

PhD. Not that kind of doctor. Sorry. Even with this degree, I don't think I'll have practical advice for her either. Maybe some comparisons to the United States about what nursing homes are like there, where my own grandmothers spent their final years, and where Charlie, a nurse, has worked in the past. How people pay for long-term care there or can't afford to. How social and racial inequalities are baked into the system there too. It's all sort of different.

Or sometimes not so different.

"That's exciting, neh! We don't get people like you around here so much. Mr. Manana comes. He's a lecturer"—another title for professor here—"he brings students from the nursing school for observations and practicals. They won't get to do a geriatric specialty at the hospitals, so they learn a lot here. Even me, I'm not a sister"—another title for nurse here—"but I learn a lot from them!"

"And here's my card," she offers, lifting from her stack in return for one of mine I've handed her. "My last name, you pronounce it the French way." She rolls the "R" like a revved engine. "Pat, my husband, was from the Congo. He had another name for me, but I won't say," she blushes. A diamond wedding ring hugs her finger. I can tell she's seen that I'm not wearing one.

"This place's different than other homes around here, so they told me," I say. Last week I dropped in to two others nearby, more upscale, where the managers told me flatly that Grace had more black people living in it.

"We're an integrated facility," she beams. "We don't discriminate. We're one big happy family!"

~

I wonder what that means—integration in South Africa after apartheid. They can't discriminate anyway—legally at least.

"Being integrated means we don't want to separate people," Angel begins. "We put our Alzheimer's patients with the others. Those patients all live in A wing together, but they eat together with the rest of the residents and move where they want. But we're careful. They don't want polished floors, and when you shower them, you mustn't start at the head. You have to start at the feet and go up. You see, they believe they'll drown. We also have the wing for pre-dementia patients—B wing. They cannot bathe by themselves, so they must wash with the caregiver. They each get a nice terrace or window, and they're free to move around as well."

C wing is for those who can do everything themselves, at their own pace.

So, integration today means keeping people together who would normally be kept apart—at least due to different care needs—and letting them move with freedom. They can choose if they want to be together—sit, chat, eat—or not.

Or?

"Being integrated also means we don't shut out the patient in need," she continues. We did see that in their mission statement out front. "The social workers call the needy ones Group Three, which just means they need assistance. We are more like a public or welfare facility, not like the nice ones you visited before. In here, you get the room, the meals, the activities, the round-the-clock help, and the nurses treat you. It used to be 6,000 rand (about $330) per month, but we've had to go up to a bit,"[1] she adds, looking unnerved.

"Most of our clients"—switching from calling them "patients"—"use their grants to pay for part of it. Of course, only if you have the ability, you'll pay the full out of pocket. That usually means your kids or the family pays. Usually tannie had a pension from her husband's job"—meaning the women here were housewives rather than wage earners in their own right—"but most will use their grant."

Older person grants are the benefit to every South African citizen sixty years and older. Like Social Security in the United States, they make or break you.[2] Here, you can get up to 2,180 rand (about $118) per month, or 2,200 (about $119) per month if you're over seventy-five.[3] Out of some 59 million South Africans total, about 3.9 million get one of these grants.[4] Intended to support a single older adult, the grants often support whole multigenerational households in black communities. Rent, school fees, electricity, water and car bills, hair appointments, personal upkeep, whatever is needed. Besides older person grants, millions of older adults can also receive child support and foster child grants and disability grants.

In the United States, the Republican threats to end Obamacare, Medicare and Medicaid, and Social Security for some benevolent yet unexplained alternative haunt us each election cycle. Both there and here, ending state assistance and social welfare for older adults would be both political suicide and a humanitarian catastrophe, I think.

And actually, I take back what I said earlier, that it "doesn't matter who you are, you have to wait." It's not the same for everyone.

Once a month in, around, and outside any of more than 1,700 mostly rural, black-majority community centers, schools, and other municipal sites, hundreds of people will stand for hours, exposed to the elements, to get the cash payouts of

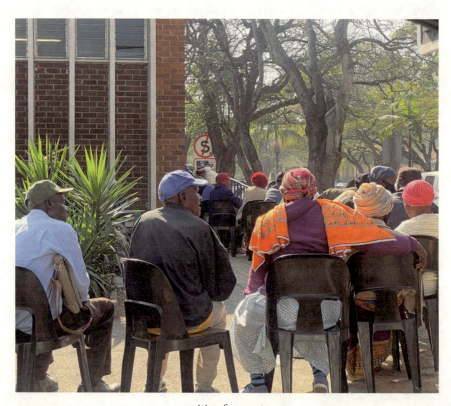

waiting for grants

their grants. This means it is mostly older people, their grandchildren, and people living with disabilities who wait in one of the most unequal economies in the world.[5]

The grant queues are legendary. The government declared "a war on queues" in 2018, promising to update pay systems by streamlining online operations through biometric screening and issuing guidelines on how to humanely manage the waiting crowd.[6] Of the 11 million citizens receiving grants of any kind, 10 million can now skip the queue to get theirs by direct deposit, accessed by a gold ATM card used wherever Visa and Mastercard are accepted. Most gold card holders are not elderly.

Entire markets of vendors, like the roadside gogo who we met earlier, grow up around the queues. What's leftover can be spent on their wares. If you didn't bring anything to eat while you wait, there are plenty of snacks for sale—roasted corncobs, fried fat-cakes (donuts), boiled nuts, macadamias. Nearby, loan sharks usually wait for their now-flush debtors.[7]

After the one-day carnival is over, the waiting crowd goes home and reconciles their receipts. It's back to life as normal, slowly spending the little amount on things that increasingly cost far too much. Inflation is everywhere. Living, aging, and dying are ever more expensive.

Everyone waits and then moves along, just not at the same pace.

"You know," she explains, "I'd say 80 percent of our clients actually come over here from the more upscale homes because they can no longer pay. It is too expensive. Like I said, 6,000 here month versus 15,000 there"—around $330 versus $850. "Some here will also get a bed subsidy, meaning government gives us money for their bed. We have forty-six beds total and five are completely subsidized, versus the two out of eighty at others like Herfseikel."

Herfseikel is a nearby upscale old age home named for nuts. In Afrikaans, it means "autumn acorns." The other nearby upscale competitor is named Macadamia.

"Some people get support from donations or funds we raise ourselves. We make money from golf events, sewing, and selling clothes and goodies"—the teddy bears and potholders in the waiting room—"baking cakes and making pancakes. People love them! We just raised 60,000 at our last event. Those pancakes sell!"

Me, smilingly: "Don't tempt me!" Again, I wish that I had had more than just coffee this morning.

"Goes nice with guava marmalade," she adds, "We make that too and sell it out front."

I cross my legs to stop my stomach from growling—"Those other homes around here, what's your relationship like with them?"

"Well, I like to say we are God's waiting room. People really need frail care and hospice options"—in contrast to long-term care for those who are not yet frail or dying. "People can try to stay active and busy on their own until they can't. The families and managers at other homes are always calling me asking if there's room for the frail ones. Those places look nice with their new buildings, but it's much too expensive to stay while you're still fit and can bathe yourself. They want to step down from that kind of place because it costs too much when there's too much time left. If we weren't so generous, we would lose more people too."

So, integration in South Africa today means accommodating people across the class spectrum—upper, middle, lower—as they all share the same fate. Before the end, they can also now live together because each pays as they can, with a little helping hand.

Or?

"You need a heart, but this is a business," she says matter-of-factly.

"I believe it."

"You know, this place has changed so much in the past couple years. It's more about the money these days. Riaan, our old CEO is gone. He was a saint to me, but I think some people hated his guts. His friend built all the little cottages here you saw driving up"—independent living units—"our big expansion, but there ended up being some problems with the construction. We couldn't build on part of the grounds because of the graves, and . . ."

"Graves?"

"It was a long time ago," she pivots. "We found a few when they did the foundations."

The cleared field of scrub grass, the wooden stakes out front near the security gate—not as empty as I thought. The stakes seemed too inadequate to be proper grave markers. But, whose graves, whose families? More unspoken questions cascade in my mind.

"The expansion problems were less about all that really. We've sorted that whole affair by now with the families. Sort of."

How do you "sort of" sort out graves under an old people's subdivision, I wonder. I've seen *Poltergeist*, and I know enough about land claims in this country to know it's never really sorted out even after the courts render their decisions: on whether historical evictions have been proven unlawful, on who has rightful access and security of tenancy, or on restitution, all what political scientist Dineo Skosana calls "grave matters,"[8]

Legal means for bodily resurrection, hopeful means for liberation.

"But," she pleads, laying the topic to rest for now, "it's not Riaan's fault, I say. It was the crap contractor. He ended up costing us millions. We're dealing with the fixes and paperwork. But still the cottages help to make us a lot of money. The market is down, and we had to get brokers to help sell a few—1.35 million rand each."

Grimace—my reaction to hearing any housing price these days as it's unaffordable to live anywhere you look. Not doing the conversion, I ask, "Is it good?"

"It's very good!"—now doing the conversion, about $75,000 for a one or two bedroom with one bath—"of course you've got admin fees and levies each month, but you also get five free days of hospice with us in the frail care here should you need it. We do the gardening and fix the pipes and other external things that we insure. They don't get title deed because it's on our grounds."

She does the arithmetic for me on a notepad with a pink pen and deck-of-cards sized calculator, sharing the actual total sales price and monthly costs with me.

"I miss him. The new CEO is a . . ."—she gives me *that* sort of look—"pushing too much on us, new rules, trainings, Zooms. For him it's all about financials. It's missing the human part, the heart. That part is important for me, the old people, and what we are doing day-to-day to keep going. I was trusted to do this job. Let me tell you about the way he shot down my bus."

I think I've seen this movie before too—Sandra Bullock? *Speed?*

"I found a man selling a big double-decker bus, so I bought it and parked it in the yard. I had plans to make it into a nice spot for the old people to sit, visit, with a small coffee shop to sell the pancakes and things. We have to rent a bus anyway to take the old people out for fun, to Kruger for safari and things. The new CEO came and said, 'You can't park that here! It doesn't belong.' It was bad. We had a woman with us who was doing, the . . ."—she Google Translates the word on her desktop—"marketing. She had said we must step it up with more fundraising. Pancakes are good but not good enough. So then, you know the rugby club in town? They took it away and shined it up like I'd wanted. There went my plan."

"You have to have the knack for business," I say. "I don't."

"It's a language you must learn to speak. Pat was in sales. I didn't know an invoice from a statement when I started here. He helped me."

Someone is going to need to help me with Afrikaans here, I can already tell from the signage and Google Translating.[9] Most of the residents prefer to speak it, she says. It's a creole language borne of seventeenth-century African-European-Asian settler-colonial and enslavement encounters here. It's also long been known more as a white language, along with English, for being promoted as *the* language by the whites in power for much of the twentieth century. It sounds Dutch and German to me—van der this and that.

"Oh, but that's wonderful that you do speak siSwati or Zulu though," she says after I explain I've studied and used those a lot instead.[10] "I never learned it."

"It"—black African languages in total, I guess she means. What most black South Africans speak as their first languages or generally know.

"Like I said, we take in everybody at our doors. Right now, we have two African women. Jane "Mama" Zulu, and Miss Motsa, who came from the streets. Motsa was just abandoned, and we brought her in. This is her home now. And we have Mr. Xitangu. He was just dumped at the hospital. No one came for him. Maureen did—the social worker. She brought him here. Now he is happy. He smiles a lot. We don't turn anyone away," she reiterates, "black, white, purple, pink—everyone's here!"

Colorful, yes, but let's do the math again. Three black people in three of the forty-six total beds she mentioned. Assuming no one is really purple—I'd be suspicious of how good the nurses are here if they were—the rest are white.

"And most are women, yes. They live longer than their husbands. I'd say it's 70/30 split of tannies and the old men. And the staff are all ladies, yes, the sisters, the kitchen ladies, the caregivers—well, except Bethal. The security are all ladies now, too. The families feel safe when they come to visit and see ladies at the gate, so I had the company staff it that way. But you see, man, woman, purple, pink, it doesn't matter. At Grace, we're like a family."

So, integration in South Africa today means that whatever your race, language, gender, sex, class, ability, or age, you are one colorful part of something bigger. Looking through the home's fence from the outside, it does appear sort of diverse—black and white, younger and older, women and men; multilingual, I'm hearing—playing the roles of people somehow related to each other.

I wonder, though, if this tour we're about to take will be a performance that Angel's somehow casted and directed, a passionate play to showcase the facets of integration she's just explained. I wonder what happens if people don't play their assigned role very well or forget their lines, or if they just improvise. The director will need to make some cuts or show 'em the door. Maybe staying on script, rather than improvising, is the price one pays to be a colorful part of that something bigger: a rainbow.

~

The rainbow, a bright arc of color, was used and meant to embody an ethos of inclusion to mark the transition period from white-minority to black-majority rule at the end of apartheid. To change the country's white nationalist image to something that honored the historically hyper-diverse, architects of statecraft, marketers, and PR firms branded South Africa as the Rainbow Nation after Anglican archbishop Desmond Tutu elaborated the term in the early 1990s. Tutu championed this ethos, chairing human rights abuse enquiries, calling for church inclusion of gays and lesbians and female clergy, and mediating between black political factions.

Years later, the archbishop visited Harvard's Kennedy School to give a speech. My Zulu class of myself, three other students, and our professor, Dr. Zoli Mali, sang Tutu's national anthem for the event. Looking back at the video, still somewhere on YouTube, I also needed a haircut. In front of the hundreds of dignitaries, ex-senators, lobbyists, and students aspiring to be such, we trembled moving through the verses, several revised in the transitional years to include the country's diverse languages.

In an inclusive change for languages at least, the new government established eleven as the official total, including the warblings of Afrikaans and English we're working through in Angel's office today. Even then, some were not deemed "official" in status—Hindi, Portuguese, Hebrew, Arabic. Today there are twelve, with sign language added in 2023.

Names changed all over the country too, for streets, parks, and whole cities—Nelspruit became Mbombela—others changing back or newly changing to black African, Indian, and coloured leaders' names or place names. The sun set on the province name of Transvaal to rise as Mpumalanga, where we are now.

In another inclusive change, on paper at least, every citizen now enjoys the same freedoms, rights, and protections from discrimination in the postapartheid constitution, implemented in 1997 and considered to be one of the most progressively liberal in the world. It begins with the statement that it's founded on the values of uplifting human dignity, nonsexism, and nonracialism. Nonracialism means rejecting ideas that scientifically distinct race groups exist and should be treated differently. Equality, as it was defined in the new Bill of Rights, meant ensuring freedom from discrimination by the state or anyone else based on their gender, sex, pregnancy status, marital status, ethnic or social origin, color, sexual orientation, disability, religion, conscience, belief, culture, language and birth, age, or race. In the United States, at the state level at least, many citizens still go without such protections.

Still, many would say that the rainbow is today nothing more than an image—vacuous, cracked, shattered, nightmarish, a fragmented performance[11]—or maybe a ghost of what the postapartheid visionaries birthed nearly thirty years ago that has since died. It is a faded image. Past to present, it never fully enchanted the white and elite minority groups in power to make substantial material changes that would empower the majority of South Africans in money, jobs, or housing.

In terms of housing under apartheid and before it, for example, the black majority lost much of their land through eviction by way of racist policies around ownership and tenure.[12] Many migrated for survival to find jobs and "squatted" on the outskirts of cities or on white-owned farms. They could be forcibly removed at any time, even after living there for generations—after building physical homes, animal pens, and gardens, and raising families and burying their dead on-site. One major documentation of the hundreds of thousands of displaced black South Africans and other people of color this happened to is *The Surplus People*.[13] By the end of apartheid in 1994, more than 10 million citizens were considered homeless or living in unserviced squalid conditions, including hostels, densely congregated building complexes for migrant laborers and their families.[14]

The new black-led government inherited this morass and implemented a Reconstruction and Development Programme (RDP) for socioeconomic uplift for black citizens and citizens of color and the marginalized among them including women, children, and older adults. Among many things, RDP called for universal social security systems and safety nets that entitled retirement between ages sixty and sixty-five, the start of private and state pension or grant options (including the older person grant), and health-related community programs to support "the elderly."

Housing was explicitly named as a human right and linked to other basic needs like water, electricity, transportation, food, health care, social security and welfare, employment, and tenure of one's environmental surroundings. The government designed, built, and paid for what became known as RDP houses, 250–350-square-foot, single-family homes for those who earned between nothing and 3,500 rand (about $240) per month. Besides income eligibility and other criteria related to citizenship and veteran status, "single aged persons without financial dependents" qualified to receive one.

Millions of RDP houses have been built since the 1990s. But by the 2010s, developers' lack of progress, abandonment of projects, poor construction, title deed issuance, and extralegal use and sale of RDP houses mired the program. This, in part, led to a rise in housing-related social movements, new political parties like the Economic Freedom Fighters, and state rectification programs to shore up public confidence.[15] In a rebranding effort, RDP houses became BNG houses—for "Breaking New Ground"—and increased to 430 square feet in size to include two bedrooms, an open living and kitchen space with a sink, a bathroom with toilet and tub, and electrical hookups.

Still, wait times are notoriously long for BNG house approval and eventual construction by a subcontracted developer. Some wait years and never see a home materialize. Many black citizens, including older adults, those who fought against apartheid, must wait for a place to live.

The illusory thing about a rainbow is that it's also based in whiteness. According to physics, white apprehends all the colors we may see in rainbow. A rainbow becomes visible to us mostly when undifferentiated white sunlight strikes through water droplets of rain, fog, or mist. Optically, when we see a rainbow in front of us, it's made from light rays originating behind us. Within a droplet, the light reflects and refracts at multiple angles. Without those vital elements—light, water, a landed vantage point—we miss the possibility for a rainbow. We're awash in whiteness.

But as something opaque blocks the light, a veil or wing, a hand covering a brow to obscure its brightness—*ukwakumkanya*, as Hugo ka Canham and others here say[16]—we begin to see shadows, a graying.

We also see gray in other mortal geneses or changes,
Like the in the depigmentation of hair and skin melanin as we age.
In the scaling pallor, colors leave.

~

"If anything, this place—all those who've gone, all the people who've lived here—teaches me that I can go quickly, at any time. Life cannot be taken for granted," Angel sighs, her nails tapping the diamond in her ring. "It's been one year and one month since Pat's gone. We were sixty and sixty-one then. From when it first happened to when he got sick, it was just three months. He had COVID, but it was all because of the "—she Googles again—"histoplasmosis. It's from a fungus he caught in the caves. Those big ones up north of here."

I remember seeing brochures for the place at the Airbnb.

"We like to travel. We spent hours in there. Stalactites and stalagmites"—like the towering binders on her desk—"all covered in kak"—bat guano—she blushes again. "It's so white, you can almost see it without flashlights. When we went home, he had breathing troubles. For a week, neh! We looked and looked online for what the problem was and read about the fungus. We thought, maybe it was in the kak . . ."

"Maybe!" I say, too encouragingly—she already knows what *it* was.

"We went to his doctor who had no idea what we were talking about. He listened, though, and did the chest X-ray. And there it was, a small hole in the lung. They took a small three-inch piece of the lung and did a biopsy."

Waiting for results can be the hardest part—before diagnoses, a name for the thing.

"We knew what it was then. I just knew. But, we went on with life," she hiccups. "The next month we went to Zanzibar, see?"

A framed picture next to the desktop centers them, two sunned-pink figures in a tropical shoal—a perfect blue beach, far from here.

Me, also sighing: "It's beautiful."

"I will never forget it. The waters, the forest. It will be with me forever. When we came back, not three months later, we were sick—COVID."

"It happens just like that," I say. Mom and Dad both got it, prior to the vaccines, in late 2020. Mom went to the hospital for kidney stones, and at a follow-up appointment she tested positive. She thinks she got it there—a hospital-acquired infection? She stayed in the isolation unit for five days, hearing five people die in the next room. Dad had it worse—flu-like symptoms, not dyspnea—but stayed home.

"Pat was bad, worse than me. We went to Mediclinic"—a private facility, with medical aid from her job at Grace—"he had to stay. The hole in the lung wasn't closing for nothing. They put a pump into his back to help him breathe. I went home and was sick as a dog, and alone. My sister has lung cancer, so she couldn't even come to check on me."

"Too risky."

"She just came to the door, placed the food, and left. It's all she could do. Pat called me and said, 'My dear, you need to hire yourself a caregiver to help you.' I was so sick, it was terrible."

The diamond in the ring shimmers. I feel a chill.

"Terrible. He stayed in the hospital, coughing so much. Black stuff was coming out of his nose, out of his mouth when he coughed. It was the fungus. It was the blackness. It was terrible."

"Terrible" spills from her story like a cloud or miasma over the towering binders.

Not being there with him at the hospital, I guess she knew what it all looked like by word of mouth. Or via video call. When Charlie and his coworkers were reassigned from their units—ER, oncology—to the new COVID wards in the early days of the pandemic, gloves came off to help hold patients' phones for such calls. On some, the touchscreen could not detect a finger through latex gloves. With masks on, the face-recognition phone feature stayed locked.

Visiting hours melted into timelessness,
And the final calls.

"I resigned after that. After he died. My mind was dying," she confesses.

"You had to."

"But Riaan, the Sisters here—Noeline and Marina—they said, 'Please, don't go.' I thought about it more, that maybe it was the wrong choice. That they need me, the old people. So, I changed my mind. That was last year. But you know, I'm sixty-one now, and come sixty-five I must retire. The new CEO says so—it's our mother office rules.[17] I mean, they can bring in someone young to do something new, shake up the jar. But if they can't find someone with my knowledge, I can stay for another year."

"Change isn't easy. I think any changeover from one way of doing things to another is hard for everyone," I say.

I wonder if I'm being subtle. I'm thinking about changes in our countries— South Africa, the United States—that were upending, vast, historical. Of racial wars past and current political strife. Of AIDS, COVID, or a time after COVID hopefully, after AIDS. After political strife, after housing insecurity. Another world that is no longer frighteningly overheating.

"Pat's still here," again tapping her ring. "I'm still married to him. That's not changing. He gave me so much that I can still go on. Wherever that is. I just want to retire and get, what are they called? A camper."

"Not a bus again, for sure," I joke.

"To travel again, enjoy. And, hey," she says, her smoky eye shadow somehow intensifying, "I now have this *new* friend."

Another sexy man.

"He is sweet. Wayne. He lives down in the cottages. They are a different part of Grace, so it's not like we're breaking the rules about amorous relations between staff and residents. Only if he wants to use the hospice inside here, then we'd have to talk. Anyhow, he used to come up to my office all the time here keeping me busy and begging to do some plan for us or manage things. I mean look around! We are running fun-day trips, doing improvement projects, new showers without the bottom rim for C wing"—it supports older people's mobility, makes it less likely you'll stumble getting in and out—"Does it look like we need help? I couldn't get rid of him!"

I feel sadder for Wayne, more than annoyed. "He wants to be useful," I suggest. He was probably active for most of his life and now sits with the malaise of retirement on someone else's grounds where someone else does the handiwork.

"Oh, I know, yes. It is funny though. But he got to me. He invited me to go to the Park"—Kruger National Park. "We drove in, had a small lunch and time together. And, he told me he loved me!"

"Do you believe in love in first sight?"

"I laughed. How can you go and tell someone so quickly that you love them? Wayne just lost his wife from COVID, too, just now, after Pat—married fifty-three years. And he's twelve years older than me. He can talk of everything, really. I don't think it's serious. But I wonder then, what's next?"

Love, I guess, or something like it, or long COVID.

"*That* was hectic"—meaning the pandemic. "The government came twice to give us tests. We had ten staff and twelve residents test positive. We had nine people pass since the first year of the whole thing, but it's been a couple years. It was bad because there was no place in the hospital, so we had to keep them here. We usually take everyone to Themba, but that was full too."

Themba's a public hospital about thirty minutes away in a township, one developed in 1974 for black people who were forcibly removed from the nearby capital city.[18] I imagine tannie Marie, whoever she is in here, in her dying hour, being driven someplace she was never meant to be in the first place.

"We turned two of the rooms into COVID rooms, and two of the nurses were assigned to help those patients. Government gave us the masks and PPE (personal protective equipment). We put those things on like we were in spacesuits! I was not even allowed to go in. Me, the manager! Just them and a doctor when he came around."

"But you got vaccinated." I'm hedging my bet. We're sort of wearing masks right now.

"The government came to give us the vaccine"—AstraZeneca—"It was very orderly! They set up tables and everything was smooth. All the old people got it. Most of them wanted it, and the rest came around to the idea soon enough. It was all fine, except for one. Old Johann. Man, that one nearly died from the shot. We thought he wouldn't make it. But he did, and he's still here."

I'm on booster three or four by now. I can't remember. She didn't quite answer the question about whether she got it. Maybe she took my "you" to mean everyone. It was a choice.

There were no vaccine mandates in South Africa, just restrictive home-based lockdowns to prevent transmission. The government deemed its public facilities too fragile to face a mass patient influx. Liquor sales were suspended. Police truly policed the streets. They hauled away white women jogging outside in the ritziest parts of Cape Town's oceanside suburbs for violating curfew.

Still, some people were safer than others. In the beginning, hospital admissions were highest in older white individuals compared to younger whites, and highest among working-age people of color in South Africa. In the first wave in 2020, a higher percentage of those working age individuals were black women who were likely providing essential services, while whites and Indian and Asian citizens were able to shelter, work from home, or afford preventive measures.[19] The first wave was also when most people died in long-term care.

"A million people died in the U.S.," I say, hedging again.

"We've always been wearing the masks here, though. The blacks were very good about it in general. They wore them all the time, like it was no big concern. I wonder if they were doing it in the townships too. Because here in town, when I go shopping, I always see them wearing them."

"Kids don't mind wearing them," I say, meaning kids in general. "By us, the parents who had suspicions about the vaccine or COVID had the problems, but kids don't complain. At least teachers and my friends with kids tell me."

32 GOD'S WAITING ROOM

"Yes, I see them playing with the masks. It's funny to watch. Look, let's start the tour and bring you to Noeline. She's our Sister of Rank. I'm going to a funeral at ten—someone who was living down in the cottages. He got to use our hospice here for the last couple days. I'll be back before lunch. It's a good one today" (again, gassing the "r")—"trout!"

~

Something about the security cameras in her office makes me bring my backpack with me, just to be safe.

From the office, back into the dining room which abuts the sitting room—the *voorkamer*—we move onto a long, long hallway, mesmerizingly long, or else the lighting gives that impression.

She strokes the faces of those we pass—"hello, hello" in a sweet childish voice, to which the faces coo, or say "goeie more."

"You see, we are just a big family in here."

"No complaints," says one man we pass.

"Eugene, this is Casey."

The man whose dark hair shines unusually due to a deep slant in his parietal bone holds a blank piece of paper the size of a Post-it.

"Hello!" he says directly. From her breast pocket, she withdraws the pink pen. Against the wall, she writes:

"My name is Eugene, I am fifty. I live in Grace, Room 2, Chief Makhaba Street. Today's date is . . ."

"What's the date today?" she blurts.

I can't remember, actually. I believe it's Monday.

"We give him one of these every day. He's been here for six years since a motorcycle accident. When I first started, he was like a vegetable. Today he's very well adapted, sociable. It's just the memory's no good. Mostly his age and the date. I think he used to be in some special unit of the police," and down to a whisper, she adds, "His roommate Louw used to laugh at him, saying his wife's gone off screwing someone else now that he's gone. What an ass."

No date needed, I guess.

"Here you go, Gene."

Three fingers receive the info. The other two are missing. He looks it over. "Didn't know that," he says with a quick review, and another "no complaints."

And then, arriving at the nurse's station, we meet her: Noeline.

"Here she is, Sister Zaayman."

"You're too young to be a doctor," the sister laughs.

Not that kind of doctor, sorry.

The towering woman with red hair, gold-frame glasses, and a military-like uniform hugs me.

"She's head nurse. We are so lucky. You know, she was Nelson Mandela's prison nurse."

"The first Sister of Rank to work on Robben Island," Noeline adds.

I'm stunned.

"You'll be in good hands here and learn a lot," Angel says, patting her hand on the nurses' station desk. Noeline's by our side, along with a crew of eight black women and one man, looking ready and less than bright-eyed for the morning shift to start. "Just be free to talk with the people. They will love you. And write the book about how we are the best old age home in the country!"

I hope.

"I have much to do today, that funeral, the diversity training, etcetera, but you'll find me around. Everyday there's something new in God's waiting room."

"Wait," I say, "before you go, what advice would you give to someone who finds themselves here? That they must come to Grace?"

I'm not so specific about what I mean by it—advice for someone who's facing aging, death, or the end in a place like this, with a new kind of family. Maybe it's a badly written interview question, or rather a good one because it's open-ended.

"Or, maybe I can ask, 'What matters in the end?'"

Angel, smiling earnestly, and looking straight into my soul: "When you age, there's always pain, but in death, you no longer feel that. Life carries on."

Heartsore

Life carries on, so she says.

Its daily starting line is the night-to-morning shift changeover—me, Noeline, another white nurse, and eight black staff members in a small huddle at the nurses' station desk, ready to run the race.

The interior design-scape of fluorescent lights and greige linoleum, plus the cool lull of the aircon makes it feel like you're half asleep inside a cloud, lying still. But:

"Oh *fok*, is it hot in here!"

A rude awakening. Her gold name tag says Janice, the other white nurse with a cropped haircut. Broad and weathered, she looks like she's had lifetime of wrangling cattle or harsher patients than the ones who live here. She lets off a few more unspeakable zingers that would make the saints cry and puts the other staff in stitches. Behind her, the electric kettle starts to squeal in the kitchenette.

Changeover starts with a song and a prayer.

"Alright. Alright! *Thula wena!* (Shut up!). Who's going to start us off," she yelps. "Goodness, c'mon now."

"*Hhayi* (No), Sis' Janice," squeaks one of the staff members, a short woman with a curly, purple-tinged wig. Being called out to lead leaves her laughing at the possible humiliation and flashing a shorn tooth from her widening smile.

"Jesus, OK. Linda, help us," Janice pleads with another woman.

"Shhhhh. Please, ladies," says Noeline, then looking apologetically at the one male staff member among them, "Let our hearts be still," trying to bring us all into the spirit.

Linda, twenty-something with braids, accepts:

"*Sizohamba naye!*" (We will walk with Him!).

As in the heart of an African American spiritual, the little nurse choir responds to her call. They've definitely heard this one before.

"Wo, wo, wo!"

"Sizohamba naye!"

"Wo, wo, wo!"

HEARTSORE

"Ngomhla wenjabulo, sizohamba naye!" (On this day of joy, we will walk with Him!).

Everyone trundles along to the hymn in a key that wavers in D. Noeline and Janice know most of the lyrics, or mouth them well at least—in siSwati, Xhosa, or Zulu, the lyrics would be the same—thank God for them there aren't clicks in this one.

Grace is near the former KaNgwane—the former native reservation and home-land for black people the apartheid government expelled from nearby towns and farms and decided were "tribally" Swazi. Also nearby is the Kingdom of eSwatini, about an hour's drive away. Until recently, its name was Swaziland until its abso-lute monarch, Mswati III, changed it. Most of the black staff come from either of these places.

Janice's swears subside. The song and a freshly poured cup of tea briefly fill her with serenity. That or she's tired, ready to head home after leading the skeleton nightshift crew of herself and two caregivers, who've already left. Someone's on duty here 24/7.

The crew's uniforms are immaculate—tailored shoulders with epaulettes, sleeves with cuffs, blouses, a burgundy color scheme today. All sharper than normal med-ical scrubs. Linda wears an enamel pin that signals higher rank. Noeline has sev-eral. Janice looks cozy in her fleece pullover.

In the huddle at the station desk, we do a methodical rundown for each resi-dent who lives here: the three black client-residents of Jane "Mama" Zulu, Miss Motsa, and Mr. Xitangu that Angel told us about and forty-one white others. Most are still in their rooms, snoozing. Some we'll meet soon—"now, now" as people say here.

The details of each one's life, its quality, or lack thereof, are handwritten in a big red binder called the Kardex. Older nurses would know it. Charlie tells me he's heard of it but never used one in his decade-plus career as a nurse. It's the older, daily record-keeping system that lists each patient's allergies, medication, care plan, and overall condition. They've been a standard in long-term care facilities. Technological creep means that most places in the United States now use elec-tronic medical records—EMRs. "Epic" is the king record-keeping system for hospi-tals and nursing homes there. Paper here.

Janice leads the rundown, the binder pages marked in blue-pen scribbles. A few acronyms and phrases get used over and over, I see, as we sweep the pages—BA ("bowel action"), SW ("slept well," her own shorthand invention). Overall, there are fewer words written down than what she tells us aloud about each resident. Because it's Monday, "there's a lot to cover" after the weekend.

We're off:

"Jane O., still critical. There's no more oxygen in the tanks that belong to us. I don't know what happened, we just filled them and they are empty already. It costs 500 rand (about $45) each to refill. We're going to have to do another training on those things, checking the pressure gauge and such. Lucky for her she's already got her own tanks. We have to watch for those."

"Jane B., still dealing with the sore on her foot. There's pus, and the bandages must be changed. The foot is fine with her takkies (sneakers) on, but once you take them off the sore starts to ooze again. It needs pressure, I think."

The last Jane—Jane Zulu—both BA and SW.

"Joan O."—not to be confused with Jane O.—"has sore shoulders. We rubbed them with ointment and some ice to dull the pain. She complains she's constipated. We gave her dried peaches and Dulcolax, but she just left the tablet by the bed, 'in case she needed it.' Woman, you do! We helped her up and took her to toilet but no BA. Then her son came on Sunday to take her out to eat"—rolling her eyes, to Spur, the steakhouse franchise. "We asked her to go before she went, but she didn't. But when she came back, she had a big one. It comes and goes with her," Janice ends triumphantly. "Maybe we'll put a commode in her room."

Noeline intercedes: "There is a reason for this behavior, and this is also a learning moment for some of you and a refresher for others. For some of these tannies, they are unsure of what is happening to their bodies. They will try to hide their incontinence and other things because they are upset or uncertain. We pay attention as nurses and notice because we are in charge of them every day. If you notice, tell us. Then we must have an intercession, reassure them that we understand. There are plenty of others just like them who are feeling this same way. They must know they are not the only ones it is happening to."

I'm struck. It's generous as an instructional point for the staff to think about why someone might be incorrigible—it might be a personal problem we can solve interpersonally. My day job is being a professor. I can tell she's a good teacher, or wants things to have order.

Other visitors like Joan's son make it into the Kardex.

"Mims's sister's daughter came to visit," Janice continues, "told us she was thankful that her aunt is smelling and looking as good as new. It's not always roses here, so mark when we do something good and get the recognition. She likes you for getting her sorted like that, Goodness, thank you."

"Aww shame," says Goodness, looking around proudly at her colleagues.

"Eunice went to the doctor with her church friend but didn't go to church. Odd. They went to Rob"—Rob Ferreira, the district's large and much-maligned public hospital named for a local apartheid-era politician and property developer. "She was flippin' mad. Her friend said they demanded she get cataract surgery, but they were turned away. The wait was too long."

"Howie went out with Tony from his church to check on his SASSA card"—the one to get his grant—"he forgot the PIN, I think, but we have to make sure that's kept safe. With the new meds, he's not shaking so much. He still has the dandruff. I'm reading the nursing guide that says normal shampooing is not going to alleviate it, so we might need a prescription."

On Sunday, three other ladies "went to church and back" with friends:

Mariejkie (sounds like "Marie-key," Little Marie)—neck pain, but doesn't want to take pain medication.

Annejkie (Little Anne)—redness on her right breast but doesn't want it looked at.

Joannettejkie (Little Little Joanne)—emotional, her sister diagnosed with leukemia.

We run by three more:

Miss Motsa—talks a lot at night to no one.

Yvonne—chafed legs; change her dressings twice per day.

Andrew—itchy skin on his back shoulders; Allergix thrice per day.

Then there are room troubles. These need a sort of tag-team effort among the nursing and housekeeping staff, rather than straight treatment mandates from those with health care credentials. Care is also about cleanliness. Two other black women staff members, also in sharp-looking burgundy uniforms, do the morning mopping behind our team huddle.

"Johnny says he sleeps at night but he's moving around in his room. You can hear his slippers slapping! Johann is probably up all night because of it"—his roommate, the one who survived the vaccine. "And I don't think he always stays in his room either. He likes to visit Mims. She's nosey and always poking around in everyone's room, so those two are meant to make trouble. Johnny's naughty, *ons boks mekaar!*" (we're always boxing with each other!).

"Mrs. Blount (Nettie) refused to bathe, but she's OK. The problem is that she doesn't want us to go in her room. It's difficult to tidy up. She's clever and you can't simply go in because she won't let you. We have to make a plan to take her down to the TV or outside to the gate, and then someone can go in and clean up. We just can't just leave it unclean in there."

"Mrs. Barragwanath ("Barra" for short) has the same sort of thing. She doesn't mind you going in but claims that nappies are disappearing from her room. Even with those doors and windows shut and locked, things still go missing, she says. Bethal (the male staff member among us) was here Friday and found six forks and spoons from the dining room in there. It comes and goes with her too!"

Noeline sounds off, recoloring Barra's case as worse than Janice says it is: "I am going to sort out her nappy story once and for all. She's always screaming that we gave her zero when we gave her four and she doesn't use them. She threatens to phone her sister to get her out of here. I am going to go in and talk to her about this. Me alone," she commands. "It costs too much to give her those for nothing, and her size is expensive. Her memory's not so good."

Last are the new ones—Mayer, Wilson, and Marais. They all moved in last week, which means some long-timers are also getting moved around.

"Mayer has dementia and we put her in A wing with LaRoux. Day 2 and we already wrote down that she's a wanderer. She's not even on any meds. Precious is starting to call her 'church girl' and 'woman of God' because, man, that woman likes to talk about the Word."

"Amen!" says Precious, the young black woman near me wearing a black tam beret and black jersey with a single pin of rank.

"And LaRoux," Janice tsks. "Poor Anne, her short-term memory's nonexistent. Mayer's good for her, because when she gets disoriented, she just talks and talks and it calms her down. LaRoux still gives us issues. You have to force her to go to bed. It's a heartsore."

"You have to beg on your knees!" laughs Noeline.

"And Marais is now with Trish," says Janice, "and she already got picked up by her son on Sunday to go out. He says he works to late in the afternoon and can't pick her up until then. Then, she came back very late. There are going to be problems with that," she ended, tapping the visitors' book.

Angel explained in the office that they've had problems when visitors don't write check-in or check-out—a case of the missing tannie, potential security issues.

Looking at the open page, Sarie Marais's son's name, first and last, is the same as the guy who's renting out his backyard cottage to me as an Airbnb. Sometimes they call these cottages "granny flats"—just coincidence, maybe, that this Sarie's here and there's an empty flat for someone like me to rent.

The rundown hits the finish line. Janice gives a few more details to the caregivers, while Noeline explains the pecking order: "We're set up in rank. There's the manager and then two professional nurses—me and Marina—but she's coming in later. I lead. We're at one staff nurse now, Janice, although we are hiring a second one soon, I hope. Jackie passed away in September, five years here. That was another heartsore. Precious and Linda here are our auxiliary nurses. The rest are caregivers, but they have certificates—Goodness, Bethal, Gugu, Yolanda, the other angels you see here—maybe you call them nurse aides, or something else. They are brilliant. We just don't have the payroll to hire so many at the next level. We can't do our job without them."

"Aww shame," says Goodness again, along with a few others' coos and "aww"s.

"We do our job but need the consult to do the best we can sometimes. Unless the resident has their own doctor, we have doctors come from the public hospitals to consult. We've got Dr. Bronkhorst for psychiatric, and another one, Dr. Chungu, an African doctor, and his wife is a psychiatric practitioner. They're a power couple! There is even a Canadian who does some short-term consults here when he's on safari at the Park. They all usually give referrals for Themba, or if they need psychiatric services, they go to Rob in Nelspruit. Oops, I mean Mbombela."

The two signs we saw on the road. Different names for the same place.

"We do need to grow with them," she instructs. "The people voted for this government, and they give the people what they want. It is their past. It is their place too."

Janice wrinkles her face, yawns.

"We have very good support from the public hospitals," Noeline continues. "Before COVID, we could just call them up and drive them over. Now we call and wait for them to tell us to come or not. The doctors there have a lot of our people on file. They know their history."

"Oh fok!"

"Janice, my *vrou* (lady)! What's the bother?" laughs Angel.

The manager's just floated back into the station with a dozen white balloons. "Surprise!"

"Oh c'mon now, everyone sing!" Noeline commands.

Janice looks like she's going to hurl.

Unlike this morning's hymn, this one's in English—the "Happy Birthday to you!" verse times four.

"Fifty-nine years. Pure gold!"

"Not a day over forty-five," says Linda.

Up from behind the little nurse choir comes Theresa, Janice's daughter, a baby with pierced ears on her hip and dragging a curly blond boy of about two who's wearing a lime green lizard-hooded pajama suit. The trio faithfully picks her up after every shift so she can babysit while Theresa's at work.

"OK, Janice, now's the time to get a new man," Precious pokes, "a boyfriend at least." Ron, her ex, has been out of the picture for a few years.

"C'mon, man," barks Janice.

Theresa: "I'll find a new one for her."

"Once a woman gets her kids from her husband, that's it. She should get divorced!"

The caregivers squeal, laughing at Janice's call to be a single-mother independent woman.

"What in the world? Don't be so negative, hey," says Angel.

"We don't need them," says Janice. "They just make our lives more complicated. A mess!"

"Alright, neh," the manager obliges, seeing she won't win her over. "See you later."

Bethal carries up a box-tray of cupcakes—yellow-white iced.

"Carrot," sighs Theresa. The lizard boy's mouth is smeared with sweet detritus.

"Save them for tea," says Noeline. "Let's go to it, by the grace of God."

Another box gets passed up from behind: plastic smocks. Like Kleenex, filmy sheets exude from the perforated hole. The caregivers each pull one out. Over head and shoulders, they veil their sharp outfits in thin plastic. Coverage for the anticipated morning messes—for waking up the residents, removing possibly soiled sheets, changing nappies, finding crumbs of midnight snacks.

These days, the mornings warm more slowly. Most residents choose to lie under their blankets, waiting for their unfurling. The season's changing.

"My son always got sick when the weather changed," says Angel.

"Same, sometimes," I reply, finding an inroad with her. "For me, it used to be hay fever."

"Like Andrew, take the Allergix," she prescribes. "If it works for the old people here, it will work for you."

I offer the recipe of hot water with lemon and cayenne in the morning for congestion, sometimes with honey.

"Oooh, refreshing! You can make that at home. Pepper, yes, if you take, or as much as you tolerate. I used to do the coconut oil regimen. I'd forget to take it or was too lazy. The coconut is memory, they say. I need it! If not, I'm going to end up in here like the clients!"

"Oh!" Angel startles. We're alone now at the desk—the caregivers gone tidying—except for a woman who's suddenly appeared beside us: LaRoux.

She says to her: "Anne, good morning," and to me: "She speaks English only. Up already, my love?"

She plants a kiss on the cardiganed woman's forehead.

"This is Casey, he's a doctor."

Not that kind. Sorry.

Anne blinks.

We wait.

"She usually asks for something. Sweets or something. We'll give her some cake."

She blinks.

We wait.

"He's here to hear people's stories. To learn who we are, where we've been, where we're going."

She blinks.

We wait.

"Anything, LaRoux? Anything?"

She blinks, testifies in a single sentence:

"I'm not afraid."

Presents

"This one looks a little fuzzy."

A single rotten cherry tomato—a strange fruit among the others that the care-givers Goodness and Yolanda hand off to me to sort through.

We're rifling through a mix of components that will make up a giant salad in a silver bowl. Not usually part of their duties, but today the kitchen's short-staffed.

Goodness shows us a WhatsApp picture of a "protest" on the road near one of the townships where a few absent kitchen staff live—a single burning car among abandoned others—over "corruption" and to call attention to things needed in the community that are still missing,

Like running water, electricity,

Safety, dignity.

"This is good stuff," says Yolanda, referring to the tomatoes. "They get it from Woolworth's."

I'd say the store is South Africa's fancier version of Whole Foods—no relation to the American Woolworth's department store luncheonettes where sit-in pro-tests for racial integration occurred in the civil rights era, as far as I know. At least I remember one historic picture of this happening at that store.

Green lettuce, spinach, avocado, cherry tomatoes, carrots—the stuff we're work-ing through, looking for spots, fuzz, and other imperfections. The carrots look the worst. The tops are dirtier, remnants of stalks like the remaining scrub grass on the cleared patch of yard near the home's gate where nothing else grows.

My condo neighbors back home pay for a special service that delivers unlovable-looking fruits and vegetables in a box to their door, victuals not pretty enough for supermarket display.

The two tear the greens by hand.

"Why would you put spinach in a salad with lettuce?" asks Yolanda.

"We cook this down for dinner. You know *umbhidvo*, Casey!"—wild spinach, pumpkin leaves, other hearty dark greens that contrast to the pale lettuce—"You're going to get us fired!" laughs Goodness.

I've put too many suspicious-looking tomatoes to the side, maybe half of three large cartons.

Be less judgmental. Too many in the trash means too few in the salad and too-plain a meal. They're supposed to offer a menu to the residents that's healthy and has some colorful and nutritional variety.

"We'll just wash the good ones. They'll make it nice in the kitchen," soothes Yolanda.

"Like the trout?" recalling Angel's excitement for the menu.

Goodness squeals. "They don't make the bread either. It's donated too. My mother's in an old home too. They bake the bread every morning."

"Your mother's in an old age home?" I'm surprised. Again, it doesn't seem common, neither here with only Mama Zulu, Mr. Xitangu, and Miss Motsa nor for black communities generally in South Africa. Or so I've read and been told.

"Yah, neh, it's by where I live. I'll take you just now. Too far for Woolworth's," she scoffs—fancier grocery stores are in certain neighborhoods and not others, obviously. "They get money from Lotto."

The National Lottery—I saw the logo on a few certificates of appreciation hanging on the wall in Angel's office. Regulated gambling has long been a way to raise money in modern nation-states, especially for social welfare. The thirteen colonies in America did it, and many countries in Europe. Gambling was effectively banned under apartheid, at least in white-majority areas. The government allowed some of the black homelands to open casinos in the 1970s to give the illusion that these were indeed separate countries, in their white minds, and to raise revenue. These casinos were effectively owned by whites, too. After apartheid and the reintegration of the homelands, the new government created the National Lottery in 2000.[1]

According to Powerball, one of the global companies contracted by South Africa's Lottery, it gives 47 percent of its gambling revenue to charities. Of that 47 percent, 50 percent must go to organizations that provide, among other services, "home-based care services for ill people, the elderly, and vulnerable groups." In 2022, for Powerball, that was about 26.5 million rand ($1.5 million).[2] It's also been mired in corruption.

"What's the name of the home where you mom lives?"

"Hlayisekani. It's Shangaan."

In that language, it can mean "security."

I Google Maps it—no website—it's in a dusty-looking area, a few kilometers from the fence of a private game reserve where tourists go to look for herds of elephants.

Marina comes up behind us to confirm what we know: "Woolies sends us these yummies one day after expiry, so they are not bad yet. We love things that are free!"

She borrows me from the salad bowl.

"Look, we're in the newspaper!" she beams.

It's a little one-hundred-word column about a fundraiser and some of their sustaining donors. In the grainy pictures, I see Angel, Marina, other white women;

PRESENTS 43

white men in short sleeve shirts and short pants—no black people, nor Noeline—smiling, next to a giant stack of pancakes.

~

Last week, down a deep escarpment with a cascading river, I visited a sister home to Grace, another daughter of their same mother organization. Farther from the capital city, and farther today from the main road which was moved years ago in a major construction project,

It is in a ghost town—killed by development.

Like its neighbors nestled in overgrown yards, the home was called Silverdays and housed in a little nineteenth-century former railway station made of field stones with grand interior arches that gave it the look of an ossuary or catacombs—in the back, a bounty of cabbage and other green leafy vegetables in a garden.

Sonya, the manager there, a woman whose family immigrated from West Germany in 1968, told me they rely heavily on donations.

"What about Eskom," I'd asked. Like the National Lottery, another parastatal, the country's electricity supplier, which also gives to charity.

"Eskom only gives for old age homes when it's 70 percent black. Our numbers are the wrong way."

Silverdays had six black residents out of thirty total.

"They do give for the old people feeding scheme we run in the township school next to us, Khayalami."

In siSwati, *khayalami* means "my home." The people visit to eat there, then return to their own.

As I left that day, a young blond man, demented from a car accident she told me, came in to fetch a plate of food prepared by the Silverdays kitchen staff. Like a bridegroom, he carried a small origami-like bouquet of white paper napkins and spork, its stem bound with a rubber band. It's for an invalid townswoman who cannot cook for herself. Every day, he leaves the plate for her at the nearby liquor store.

"The people are too poor to be contributors," she said. "Baking cakes or other sweets, it's not viable because most of them cook those things in their homes and try to sell it for money themselves."

~

"I love when young people come to visit," Marina continues, "From the private school and other places. It's like another gift, a present. Some have their favorite and they talk to the same ones every time, their buddies. The younger ones also

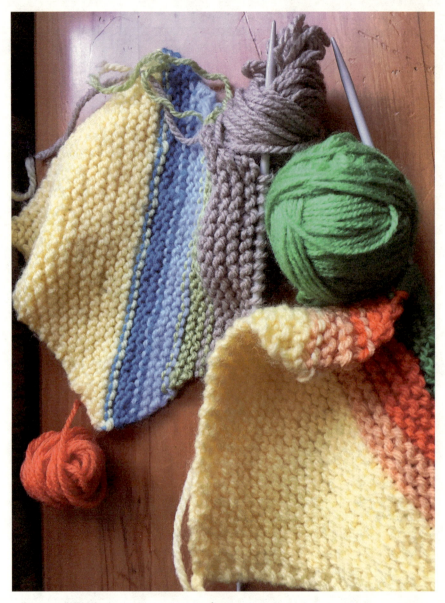

knits

come to play music in little concerts, and we take the residents to visit the schools too. Last year, we took them to Bundu Lodge for a free brunch!"

"Yum!" No mimosas, I imagine.

"Kruger doesn't let us for free, but we go in Heritage Month. Then for us they waive part of the fee!" For citizens, she means.

We walk further down C wing, stopping to meet another pair. Jane B. and Joan O. Today, they are citizens, but once they were immigrants. Jane came from then-Rhodesia with her war veteran husband. "Yvonne, my room neighbor is also

PRESENTS 45

from there," Jane grins. Joan came as a child from Sweden with her missionary grandparents.

They're knitting potholders.

"More little donations," says Marina, "scraps of wool from projects that the ladies do at church. When it's not busy, I love to help!" She looks over to the waiting room where we entered, where the other potholders and teddy bears sit softly, waiting for purchase.

"I just start making small shapes," says Joan, "not knowing what they'll become. I just try."

Jane listens, then starts to tremble. She swallows, then croaks: "God is so good. Today, I go by His strength. I see it as a gift. He's helped me out in so many situations."

"That's wonderful," I respond a bit too quickly.

"You see, there was a time I was dying. Everyone here saw me."

"It wasn't good," adds Marina, "her breathing. We took her to Themba."

"After two days in there, I just asked to die. Just finish it. But He didn't. He had a different plan for me. God has a plan for everything. If it is not your time, it is not your time; we have to go by what God says. When He is ready, then it's your time."

Jane tears a little. I feel I might too. I rub my eyes. Blinded momentarily, I only hear her chuckle,

"Yesterday is history, tomorrow is a mystery.

Today is the present, it is a gift from God."

"Ack, shame," sighs Marina.

Joan pivots to address her own challenges: "It was also difficult moving in here. I used to live down in the cottages."

"Is life in general difficult?" I ask.

Marina watches Jane reposition her knitting needles. Her hand is bandaged.

"People have their own dreams, their own desires and ideas," says Joan. "The ladies who live here, me, we did things our own way. Now, when you live with other people, you must adjust because you are not the only one. They used to be the bosses and tell others what they wanted and when they wanted it."

Heads of households, keepers of husband and children, side hustles, and, in all likelihood, domestic workers. The lady-baas.[3]

"Now, they must wait for others, rather than getting theirs first. And *they* want to get theirs too now because things are different after the change," she adds.

I know who she means. Her switch from talking about her white home-mates' daily goings-on to the country's black majority in the postapartheid freedom era is startlingly seamless.

"They still have the idea that they should get things for free. That is how it was before. And they still have that idea now, even if we are all the same after the change. My mother and father worked at a mission hospital. We spoke Zulu and Swazi. And Swedish and English, of course. You know that word they say when they come to ask for something at that time of the year? They came to ask for Khisimus."

The translation in those African languages for the English word "Christmas."[4] To someone like Joan, it means a black person asking for a present come December.

"They would come and ask us what they will get for Khisimus, expecting something for free. And you know, I wonder what it means for something to be free. I remember, when I was a pensioner, but, oh, wait I still am! I mean before living here. I remember I once I went to fill up my car. The attendant came up to me, and I said just to him, 'Where is *my* Khisimus?'"

I think we know what would possess this white woman to straight-up ask that of a man who I assume was black.

"What about me?" she pleads, rhetorically now. "Now, we are all equal. You were not free then, but now you are working, and I am no longer working as an old person. So, we are now like the same. He looked at me very confused. And now they have rights as well. That is hard for some people in here."

"Ack, shame," sighs Marina again.

On her encouraging, I explain to Jane and Joan what I'm doing here, why we want to take the tour, think about who ends up in a place like this, and who doesn't.

"Yes, the white churches built places like Grace," Joan says, "but the Afrikaners used to put us like this." She puts her hands in a prayerful position, ivory fingers tightened together, polished nails up, aerodynamized like a church steeple. Slowly, she breaks the position, sliding her hands away from each other.

"Apart?"

"I am surprised they are building old age homes out there in the townships like Goodness says," admits Marina," It's not something you see for them. The government is not providing enough."

For black people in general, or older adults?

"That is why the churches must step in," Marina explains. "Money's always needed because maintenance is ongoing. There are costs to keep everything going over time. You can't just build a place like this and then let it go. It is the same for the old people. They are happy here and content, and if they have someone in the area like family to come visit them, it is fine, just to pop in once a week. Some people, they check their family member in there and don't come back, dare I say, 'dump them.'"

Joan and Jane look blankly at her daring statement.

"The community here is also so good to them," she continues. "They bring them so much. Especially around Christmas."

Jane gives us a blessing that we learn something new on the tour. And remember,

"Yesterday is history, tomorrow is a mystery.

Today is a present. It is a gift from God."[5]

"When you get old, you give up more and more," says Marina, moving on from the pair.

"What do you give up exactly?" I wonder.

"Well, memories, I think. I'm sixty-five and it's even hard for me. For someone like LaRoux or Mayer, they struggle to remember the finer details of life. But then I think some people are just too lazy to think."

We're back at the nurses' station. Marina's got a performance review to do with a caregiver Gugu, her first-year-in-the-workplace anniversary. The auxiliary nurse Precious has accompanied her to the station desk.

Precious adds, "Sister knows. Everyone is not the same here even if you're old. Some of them do not know what is going on outside"—of the home, I guess, the general news of the turning world beyond the fence. "They might remember things from the past, but not remember what is happening today. They forget recent memories."

Some memories may be too much to go on with. Some wish they'd be forgotten or remembered differently. Their talk reminds me of "RhodesMustFall." It was a student movement that began here in late 2014, when I was working in Johannesburg. In part, it involved a push to remove statues of oppressive colonial figures like Cecil Rhodes on university campuses. He's the namesake of Rhodesia, Jane B. and Yvonne's former home, as well as Rhodes University in Grahamstown. Progressive students there call it "the university currently known as Rhodes" to signal ongoing efforts to change the name. In a 15-to-9 vote, the university's administrative council voted against the name change in 2017, citing financial constraints[6]—maybe signs for new names are too costly.

Some statues, names, and other symbols—like the Confederate flag in the United States—also conjure painful memories. They're put up by those in power to be *the* way we should remember.

"Well, I mean, that's different," Gugu responds to my train of thought. "Those statues make the cities look nice. Mandela told us in 1994 that we are one nation. They are being crazy over a statue that means nothing."

"But aren't they a sore reminder of what came before?" I try to pull in part of the word "heartsore" we've heard before.

Gugu again: "Casey, aren't there lots of other statues for blacks too? Like Chris Hani?"

Chris Hani was an anti-apartheid activist and a leader in the South African Communist Party (SACP). He received a BA from Rhodes University in 1962 and joined Umkhonto weSizwe, the military wing of the African National Congress (ANC), the same year. After being jailed for protest actions and campaigns, he left for the Soviet Union to undergo military training, returning in 1967 to join the Zimbabwean War of Liberation from white settlers claiming it as Rhodesia— like Jane B. and Yvonne. With other ANC members in exile, he convened the 1969 Morogoro Conference in Tanzania, which permitted whites and other non-Africans to join their movement.[7]

Hani continued guerrilla war tactics across Southern Africa for the next twenty years, supporting the anti-apartheid struggle from Botswana to Lesotho, Angola, and Zambia. He successively rose through the ranks of both the ANC and the SACP. After the unbanning of black political parties in 1990, the SACP was poised to play a serious role in national politics as Hani helped them gain popularity in the townships from his speaking tours.[8]

In 1993, a year before apartheid's end, Hani was shot at point-blank range and killed, in front of his wife and teenage daughter, by right-wing extremist Janusz Waluś. A public memorial to Hani was built in Boksburg's South Park Cemetery in 2015, for all to behold and remember.

Waluś and an accomplice received the death sentence. It was commuted to life in prison in 2000 after the postapartheid constitution was enacted and forbade this punishment. In 2022, Waluś, then sixty-nine, was discharged on medical parole after he was stabbed by another prisoner.

In contrast, on the same day of this discharge decision, the Supreme Court of Appeals revoked medical parole granted to Jacob Zuma. Zuma, then eighty, the former president of South Africa and former member of Umkhonto weSizwe, was to serve fifteen months in prison for contempt of court in 2021 in a trial uncovering mass corruption during his presidency. Two months into his sentence, Correctional Services, which runs the prisons, granted him the parole for an "undisclosed illness." The actual Medical Parole Advisory Board did not find his ailment warranted release, but Correctional Services overrode their decision. The Court found that unlawful.[9]

A week after these medical parole decisions—sometimes framed as "compassionate release" for ill or aging people in prison—Hani's memorial was vandalized.[10] Its lighting fixture was stolen, and a granite pillar, representing a flowering gladiolus, was destroyed.

~

Here at Grace, there are no statues or monuments to the buried ones beneath the empty patch of scrub grass down near the gate. Simple cairns have long been the commemorative practice to mark graves here, which fade into the landscape over generations. Like I thought, the markers we saw function to show where utilities lie. And to do no further landscaping over the interred.

Among the binders in Angel's office that she shared with me to read include Grace's papers of a yearslong case to claim this plot of land the graves lay within, a claim spearheaded by a black community trust on behalf of one Mr. Malopa. In Grace's paperwork, they call him *oupa* (grandpa).

The papers include a Magistrate's Court interdict application filed by Grandpa Malopa to prevent the home from starting the independent-living cottage construction project which would potentially unearth the graves. The papers also include Grace's intention to oppose the interdict.

PRESENTS   49

After these formal filings, Grandpa Malopa wrote a letter to Angel. In it, he asked to visit the graves and conduct an "inspection in loco of our claimed land," so as to pay tribute and visit their ancestors as custom demanded, "by praying and requesting guidance, direction and blessings for our future deliberations with the Mpumalanga Claim Commission, Public Works, and the Municipality," as well as Grace's mother organization, for all to behold and remember.

When they showed up at the gate five days later, Pretty was told to turn them away.

~

"Casey, it's all in their minds," someone adds with a tsk. Behind us, suddenly, it's Joan again. She has a question for Precious.

"Sisi, can you help me? It's this one, the right. It's making noise." She gingerly holds a hearing aid in her hand for her to see.

"Aww, tannie, you should ask Sis' Noeline or Marina about that one."

"There was a problem with this one before. They took us to the . . ." she struggles to find the word. "Ear doctor. When I went this week, the doctor was out and I had to make time to come back to get a new one."

Recently in the United States, President Biden signed an executive order making hearing aids available over the counter, meaning without a prescription. Some of the big-box stores—Walmart, CVS—claim the executive order will drop the cost for a pair by as much $3,000. Many people need them—30 million Americans—and more soon will as the baby boomers age further, as we all do.[11] Maybe an order like this can happen here too, part of that pie-in-the-sky NHI plan.

"Jane and me, we both wear them. Or we're supposed to," Joan winks, "but when it's just two of us in our room after dinner, we take them out. When I was down in the cottage, I would choose not to wear it because it was just me. No one to talk to."

Precious leaves to find one of the Sisters.

"It is hard to hear with them in sometimes. In the sitting room, so many of us old people are talking. It is too much."

I believe I can hear what she describes—pervasive, mind-numbing, audibly fuzzy, people talking all at once about nothing—white noise.

"I haven't used this one for weeks now,
I sometimes can't hear anything."

Andrew

"We want some meat on his bones!"

He's a bigger guy, thick rugby player–like thighs, but other parts of his legs seem to be missing.

We're on a quick break at the nurse's station—Precious, Linda, and me—scrutinizing a supermarket ad for a bag of frozen chicken, a once proud cock now disassembled in a jumble of pieces. Even at the sale price, the picture of limbs leaves a lot to be desired.

"Nothing like homestyle," laughs Precious. Homestyle, or "indigenous" chickens are ones you find free-ranging around the yard for insects, cooking-pot scraps, and groundnuts. All-color plumage, dark meat, and lean. Broilers—"white people's chickens"—are fatter, force-fed in cages, plump with antibiotics. White feathers.

Here comes another bigger guy, more than six feet or nearing two meters tall, lean, walking softly in slippers and with watery hazel eyes—Andrew.

It looks like he's about up to say something. His mouth moves to the shape of words but speaks nothing we can hear. Just a little tremor.

"Girls, are you being naughty?" he then quips.

Precious, teasing him: "What do you want here?"

Linda: "This one!"

"He's talking to Dickie!" her colleague claims.

"Oh no, man!" he scoffs.

"This one likes to talk. He talks to himself!"

"You know I like to talk, sis'. I get along with everyone," Andrew says proudly.

"He does," warms Precious, "and Dickie's always looking down on us."

"You know he's always looking, so you two best behave or I'll call the Sisters on you," he phlegm-laughs, jabbing his ring finger in our direction.

"Dickie wants to know that we are being nice to you, Andrew!"

"Ha! These girls are always nice," he winks. "No complaints. Dick never said you were nasty, girls. You're always kind to me, always."

His eyes water more, maybe part of the tremor.

50

ANDREW

The girls take off to the sluice, the methodical name for the washrooms for bodies, bedsheets, whatever needs a rinse. Just us now, and we're off to the patio, to take off the masks for a bit. For Andrew to smoke.

Noeline pops out briefly as we sit down on the wire chairs. "Darling, the ship sails on Thursday. I am begging you to come."

"Ah, Sister, please." How could she believe it would sail without him.

They mean shopping. Thursday, every other one or so, one of Sisters or Angel takes their personal car out to one of the shops—Spar, Clicks, any other with a good sale marked in the weekly ads. The residents don't get out themselves. No one has a car here. They'll pick up requests, from the random to the I-would-sooner-die-than-live-without-this. Within reason—that being the Sisters' assessment of how badly it impacts their health or not.

For a handful, men mostly like Andrew, it's cigarettes. Dunhills and Peter Stuyvesants are the most popular. Peters are proudly South African, launched in 1954, a few years after apartheid commenced. All the white nurses smoke too. They prefer Pall Malls.

For the rest, it's snacks and treats—chocolate, macadamias and other nuts, biscuits, biltong. Dried fruit—apricots, prunes—is already on hand. The Sisters keep it stocked for constipation.

Andrew, another sweetie according to Angel, always goes along. It's a treat for both him and the staff. They both like the company.

"After lunch, neh," Noeline says. She looks at me, him. Leaves.

He coughs and upturns the Dunhill.

It's only been thirteen months since he and Dickie moved in. Angel told me Dickie's been gone eleven.

Besides the itchy upper back for which Janice prescribed Allergix, he lives with epilepsy. He hasn't had a seizure, though, in four years, another on-the-side factoid from Angel. Takes his meds normally according to the Kardex, lives in A wing among the residents with dementia although not living with it himself. Dresses, grooms, bathes himself, and is not living with a noticeable debility—a problematic assumption, I know. What you can't see may be the worst. Besides all this, "no complaints." Like Eugene says.

"I tell you, those girls are cheeky, neh?"

Silly, maybe. Cheeky's too British, or too condescending—it's both, I think—even if I can tell he trusts them, and they him. Their banter felt comfortable, like ours does now. He's familiar, like someone who seemingly knows me already, or sees himself in me, somehow.

"Still, the girls, Noeline—*nobody* knows about me though, *neh*."

The lilt—as if to say, "*You* know, though, right?"—chewing his lip in an upcurled smile.

Do I?

He crosses his long legs at the kneecaps and runs his gold-ring-fingered hand over the back of his buzz cut. In a white plaid and brown stiffened-collar shirt under brown zip-collar sweater, it's a boy's Sunday best for an eighty-four-year-old.

"Oh, I bet they can be naughty when they want to be," I say, using the word he slung at the women for their jokes.

"The Sisters know I watch for that kind of thing. You don't know what some people can do, neh? Ja, no, those are good girls. They like me, and I like all of them."

"And Dickie?" I ask.

He studies my whole face in an instant. And maybe my own crossed legs. On the wire chair, he taps the unlit cigarette pinched between his thumb and first finger. Leaning in, in an almost-whisper:

"No one knows about us, I tell you."

I look at him blankly.

"You just keep quiet" or "You just keep your mouth shut," he says only by smiling. "The others, they don't understand. It's not what they believe in."

Precious, Linda, maybe Bethal—Bethal who helps the male residents here the most—all keepers of Andrew's open secret. The "others" are the tannies, the whites, his A wing neighbors with dementia who might not know him to be any different than other man they've known—their late husbands, sons, or neighbors. Someone like them in some way.

"Nobody knows about us," resounds in my ears.

He lights the cigarette.

~

Nobody knows about us.

I wonder, who or what is "us" then, when "they don't understand" or believe in that which makes us who we are?

Noeline and the caregivers see this "us," I think, in Andrew and I sitting out here among the geraniums, quietly invested in hearing each other, burnishing in fresh contact. I wonder whether he's met anyone like me, like Dickie, in months or years. Again, Grace is mostly older widowed white women and younger black staff women. And again, there are exceptions.

But this may be less of an "us"-versus-them situation. Divisions exist, yes, but dividing lines are often dotted or porous. He and I can stand nearby or nearly within a place we think we belong to and still feel somehow outside of it. Knowing that our belonging there, to any place, is based on others' misperceptions of who we are. Belonging is always evolving. It's impermanent, fretful, must be defended.

And how does someone "know" about us? And by what sense?

Do we know by seeing? Vision can be unclear too, due to astigmatism, dissonance, or your beliefs in that you "see" something differently than someone else.

Do we know by speaking, or trying to—like in Andrew's silence, in seeing lips move without speech but knowing he's saying something.

ANDREW

Or, do we know by hearing—the supposedly perceptible "gay"-sounding aspect of a voice, the question of its existence being a flashpoint for psychologists, speech pathologists, and a stereotype that also haunts many gay men. Some internalize, refute, or reclaim it.[1]

Andrew doesn't sound gay to my American ears—and all the studies about "gay voice" were based in the United States or in Europe, not here, again, where there are more than twelve languages, official or not.

His voice sounds phlegmy still from smoking, raspy from years of it. He sounds kind.

Or do we know by touch?

Depending on the translation of Genesis, chapters 18 and 19, the townsmen battering the door of Lot's home in Sodom wanted to "know" the angels being sheltered inside, or "know them carnally"—in other words, rape them. Lot offers his daughters to the men instead, but God and/or the angels intervene to blind the men. The following morning, Lot's family flees Sodom, after which God destroys it and the neighboring Gomorrah in a sulfuric firestorm. Lot's wife is punitively transformed into salt for looking back to witness the chaos. Lot finds haven in a cave with his daughters, who have sex with their wine-drunken father to renew their lineage.

Some conservative evangelical theologians take the myth of destruction, the townsmen's desire to "know" the angels, as a castigation of the Sodomites' supposed homosexuality. More liberal theologians and religious studies scholars, and even some locals here, argue that God was displeased with the townsmen's supposed inhospitality and destroyed the town because of it.[2]

Only in death, do we part this world.

But even then, I wonder, do we?

~

"He was so much to me," he says, bringing us back to Dickie.

"I know."

"We had our own room here. My bed, his bed." Grace's standard is twin-sized. "I had his picture by mine, mine by his." Noeline had helped to hang each picture above their headboards.

It was more a necessity to move in. Dickie's health was declining fast. Andrew didn't have the strength to get him into the tub and out, to roll him over and up in the night to use the toilet.

"He was sick, neh, but going on just fine. But then came January. And just one day. After lunch, we lied down. He couldn't catch his breath, making noise. To try to . . . just to try. 'Sister!' I said. I went out and got them. I couldn't . . ."

"Stay out here, just wait," Precious and Linda had told him, staying with him in the hall.

I've reached out just now to hold his hand. To touch.

"I didn't know what was happening. I didn't know what was wrong. I couldn't. I waited forever. I waited. Noeline came. She had the look in her eyes," he says, choking. "I knew."

His hand is cool, gentle, enclosing all of mine in it.

"I nearly went mad," his eyes watering again. "No, no, man. No. What can I do? What now?" he quickens and trails off.

Our hands are holding still.

When I lost someone once (not quite like this), my therapist sometimes just said nothing when I talked about it in session, just looking at me contemplatively. Or blankly. I couldn't quite tell. It forced me to keep making sense of what had happened,

To know it by speaking of beautiful things.

"We loved to go to the botanical garden, to see the waterfall. It's where we put his ashes. I was shocked at the expense—6,000 rand ($330), man! They tried to upset me with the casket. What do I need that for? I wanted simple, for the simple person who would be inside it. He never wanted for anything. He came back to me in a small box you can open like a drawer."

"Andrew," I murmur.

"We have friends who live on a farm near here. They still take me out for Christmas and other times. They took us to the gardens. So he could be there."

The cigarette smoke makes an arc from his chest, outward to Heaven as he mimics casting the ashes—love blown down to the pool amid the garden's monstera, where the waterfall ends. I've gone walking there myself on lonesome Sundays.

"Sometimes, they take me back. To visit him."

"Andrew," I murmur again.

"After that, I moved to another room. The Sisters gave me another roommate. He was fine, some bloke with nice teeth. It wasn't too long though, maybe two, three months when he passed away too. It was about one week later, and Noeline came and said, 'Andrew, you are going to get your own room. Do you mind?' I don't. I am happy to have privacy, the quiet to myself. I'm a private person."

"How did you meet Dickie?"

"His firm was across from mine"—eyeing each other from across the courtyard, one of those modernist-veering-on-brutalist buildings that defined high-apartheid architectural style, I imagine—"in Pretoria. Then we moved to Benoni. I also grew up there. We became fast friends. Never went anywhere without him."

Benoni—what is today mostly Johannesburg suburbia. The country's biggest airport, O. R. Tambo, is next to it. Originally built up between four large settler-colonial farm plots, the discovery of gold in 1887 transformed the area into a metropole within a couple of decades. After World War II, in Andrew's childhood, much of the actual farms were already overrun by new housing subdivisions, and actual farm work was managed by Goldies Dairy and then Bill Davey. Davey became Benoni's mayor and is remembered by some for "driving for the establishment of respectable housing for blacks, most notably Daveyton, in the midst of the Apartheid era."[3]

"One-, two-bedroom?"

"Three! In a complex—Bedford Gardens it was," he recalls.

"Luxury! I'll look for it when I go there next."

"You can say, eh," laughing. "Two bathrooms, kitchen, courtyard, and at the front of the lounge was the garden and swimming pool. It was our home. We were married there."

That certainly wasn't legal.

In 1961, when Andrew was nineteen, the National Party implemented its Marriage Act, a move that standardized marriage for the whole country—undoing specific laws for the five formerly separate colonies-turned-provinces of the Union—and effectively made marriage to be only between a man and woman. It also invalidated black African customary or traditional marriages previously deemed legal by the white government.[4]

The apartheid government was obsessed with regulating what went on in people's bedrooms. Previously, they'd passed the Prohibition of Mixed Marriages Act of 1949, when Andrew was seven, preventing marriage between whites and any other "race group," and the Immorality Act of 1950, when he was eight, prohibiting adultery and "immoral" acts like sex between "race groups." In 1961, under pressure for these inhumane moves and more, South Africa left the Commonwealth of Nations.

Of course, these definitions of marriage later conflicted with the postapartheid constitution which guaranteed protections from discrimination based on sexual orientation and gender, before any law like it in the United States. But still, nothing on the books here made same-sex marriages legal.

It was a lesbian couple—Marié Adriaana Fourie and Cecilia Bonthuys, two Afrikaner women—that led the way. A local magistrate acknowledged their 1996 marriage but refused to register them. The High Court, the next level up, also refused to register them in 2002. After that, advocates at the Lesbian and Gay Equality Project helped raise the case to the Supreme Court of Appeals and Constitutional Court, which ruled in the couple's favor to enact the Civil Union Act and affirm their marriage by 2006. It took ten years.

South Africa became only the fifth country in the world at the time to legalize same-sex marriage. There were local dissenters, of course, including the influential Anglican Church—the church's famous figurehead, Desmond Tutu, he supported it.

Andrew says they were married in their flat, by an Anglican priest, in secret. He was also gay, in secret. There was no ceremony. No one else was there.

(No one knows about us.)

"Our neighbors liked us though, hey. We didn't like going to parties and things, going out and about. But, wherever we went, we went together."

"What about here, though?"

"Eh, man?"

"They liked you and Dickie and . . ." I probe.

Coughing: "It is better to just keep quiet."

For a few seconds, a bird chirping nearby is the only sound we hear.

"Because you will still be married," he says, "it's just . . . no one will know."

I let it go.

Maybe we are talking about two different things, or two aspects of marriage, each of us foregrounding one part of it. Andrew, referring to marriage as a binding promise by two people to be near one another, always, a never wavering position of commitment despite being shrouded, invisibilized. Me, referring to a right, a public acknowledgment that makes the commitment something more. I don't want to say more "real," but openly recognized, at least.

I now realize we haven't heard him say anything about "love" besides their fondness for the botanical garden. Or how they came to live here, nearly a four-hour drive from Benoni. Maybe, because no one would know them out here. Maybe, being childless, this lower-cost option is what they could afford without the financial support of adult children. So much for the DINKs (dual-income, no kids).

For now, I have "goddaughters" only, girls in eSwatini who are part of families I came to know and lived with as part of a road trip I took once like this one. Girls who've grown into young women and I've supported in different ways. Otherwise, at home I have what the American Millennials call "plant babies" (houseplants), a stretch from "fur babies," the name for pets-as-children.

"We had two dogs," he laughs, "Jack Russell Terriers."

"Cute, I am sure. Do you wish that you could have pets here?" I haven't seen any animals as pets or as service providers yet.

"I do, but they think they are too loud for this place. The Jack Russells were good boys, nice to walk, and very companionate. They just knew you—what time we went to work, when we came home. They're just waiting by the door."

Somebody knows.

"I grew up on a farm," he pivots. "We kept cattle for the dairy, horses, and what are those little peckers . . . chickens. Those times were carefree, as a youngster. I liked riding my bicycle and horses. I very much loved swimming. All my life I've been brown!"

Meaning?

"Tanning in the sun when I was swimming. One day I'd be as red as a tomato, the next day, brown."

I see.

"Carefree, but they were strict"—his parents. "We were a loving family. My mother was English, always worked. She was a lawyer's secretary for many years. She loved me. After she finished work, she came home and did what she was supposed to do." I guess as a housewife, a woman of those times. "She loved people and got along with everyone. She was active in church too—Anglican."

"Like where you were married, sort of," I tease. "And your father?"

"He was an Afrikaner, a mechanical engineer. He was always traveling for work on the mines but also dams and bridges. He was the more strict one."

"And his purpose?"

ANDREW

57

"Work and his family," he answers quickly.

I wait a moment. "Was it for his country?" It's a possible detour of a question, but I want to know: Was his father an advocate for what was then the new South Africa? Rampant development as an imperative of the nation? Benoni was also an urbanizing mining hotspot, where men went into the earth to extract gold, make wealth. Black men, or, when they refused to work at certain points in this country's history, tens of thousands of indentured workers from China. Like in America's and other gold rushes. (They're all connected.)[5]

"He enjoyed carpentry."

"OK," I cede.

"He continued to work after he retired. Both my mother and father did. Not like today, where the laws say you must stop when you get to be sixty-five. He took the necessary three months off, then he was hired as a consultant until he stopped working again at seventy-five. Their companies didn't want to lose their knowledge when in retirement"—rather than hire or train anyone else like black people or new graduates. "Later, they sold the family home. They moved to a smaller one."

Like the cottages outside, and again, my parents' downsized house.

"Both of them died of old age. In their nineties, like their parents. They were never ill, never sickly, never had a problem a day in their lives."

Pure old age—a medically debated and neutralizing catch-all to write on death certificates. Most people in this country or anywhere are never so free of "problems" to die this way.

"After that, I sold their small home," he explains. "Maria retired."

"Who's Maria?"

I'm being facetious. Almost all white families of his parents' generation and his own had someone like "Maria." Even today, many black families and individuals also have someone like "Maria."

"She was from Lesotho, began working for us when she was very young. She worked for us for many years, all in all, maybe forty. She was always a kind person. My parents treated her like she was one of the family. She was a big Christian woman. Nothing was too much for her. Whatever you asked her to do, she wanted to please you, the people she worked for. She treated people with respect, and that is how we treated her too. With respect."

"Where did she stay? On the farm with you?"

"Yes, outside in a side room on the property. Her husband worked in the mines. He was often there. She had two children, a son and a daughter. The daughter became a . . ."—searching for the word—"teacher. Her son became a doctor," he says, somewhat brighter.

"Seems she was well supported then if her children could go far in school like that."

"Yes, she was very well paid," he cedes now. "She had a good salary."

Again, I wonder.

"Andrew, do you think helpers like Maria—is it like what Bethal or Precious or the caregivers or nurses do for you here?

Quickly, "No. They are not the same. They are a bit different. Many of them are very good. They work, but I wouldn't say some are very dedicated. Not like Maria or someone like her"—a domestic worker. "Some are just working because it is a job."

"For the sake of it? Some have been here a very long time." Angel told me Goodness has been here six years, for instance.

"Not like Maria. Look, neh, the nurses, kitchen girls, I get along with everyone, and I speak their language"—again, maybe "African language(s)" in general, or maybe that language where we "know" a true story about each other but don't speak about it directly. "There are some who have been here a long time, yes. The newer ones must be taught and follow in the older ones' footsteps. But even the ones who've been around the longest are getting older too. They must learn new things too."

"They learned what they knew in the past," I clarify, "maybe older ways of doing things, not interacting so much with others who are different from them."

"Yes," he says, picking up my too-obvious hint. "You mean since 1994"—apartheid's end. "It is different now for both the young and the old."

Just now, we can hear two children, girls, squabbling-giggling somewhere. Maybe someone's granddaughters visiting.

"We are now integrated. It is one nation. But it is different. Now there are whites going out with black folks and the reverse case. If you watch the youngsters, now they go to school together, visit each other's houses, go on holidays together. Their parents know each other, and they are friendly. The job situation is like that also. It *has* changed, and things will still change more."

"I think people had a lot of ideas about how it would all turn out after the change. After Mandela and the Rainbow. But then, for some, maybe it didn't turn out like they thought it would."

"I agree with you. It's going to take a long time!" he lilts. "I mean, you and me, we will be gone already and there will still be things to change. You know?"

It's true, but we're hungry for more, something more substantial *now*.

"But they must open their eyes and see what is going on *in the moment*," he emphasizes. "All these crazy things. It has to come to an end." He means the news, the general atmosphere of our lives, our existence. "You watch the news and you see all these crazy things. It's on a daily basis, man. We never used to have things like that all those years ago. Always a trial, always a murder."

"I know," I sigh. Besides the news, the last time I went to a Barnes & Noble bookstore, almost the entirety of the "Current Affairs" section was books about cold case murders.

"It's really bad, young ones going to school with knives and killing each other and teachers and lord knows what."

Or guns.

"We've lost some control. Lost God," I offer, recalling a song I heard once, putting it in terms I think many people in the United States use to make sense of our many losses. Umpqua. Newtown. Uvalde. Virginia Tech. Others you may never hear of if it wasn't your community or classroom. Your child. You.

ANDREW

"Yeah, even the teachers, man," he points out, meaning cases in the South African news of schoolteachers taking advantage of students—of women college students and their lecturers, bribery, and again, rape.[6] The students also revolt against this. Things must fall.

"I mean they both scapegoat each other because they don't know what the devil is going to happen. The youngster now telling the grownups what to do, not the grownups telling the youngsters."

Generational inversions,

Collisions,

Mirages.

"I guess you do that here too, keep the youngsters in line," I say—watching the staff, the "girls" here, whether they're being "naughty" or nice on the job.

"But . . . in a quiet way. I'm not loud about it. I was always a quiet person. Dick was a quiet person too. We kept to ourselves."

I think I understand his change in tone. "And when you think about the time in your life that you were most happy, was it with him?"

"Of all of my life, it was. And really, Casey. And really, everything went smoothly."

"As a young man, and then as professional?"—ordering his life by job, age, and thinking how smooth things could really go being white and gay under apartheid.

"It went smoothly. All of it."

"And here too?" I ask.

"I am used to death here. With Dick, it was the worst, the worst thing of my life. But . . ."—a drag on the cigarette's remains—"it doesn't get to me anymore."

An exhale.

"People here can't deal with it. They go crazy, running themselves mad up and down. They can't handle what they know's coming. You have to get used it to when you're in a place like this. I did."

"I wonder, if they could send a message to you today, your mother and father, from wherever they are now, what would they say to you?"

Thoughtfully: "To be responsible. That I should become responsible, be proper, to take care of myself and my life."

I wonder what Dickie would say to him.

I know he's watching him—no, "us"—now. Somehow.

~

Others might be watching us in this courtyard now, open to a dozen rooms' windows, where we can hear others' grandchildren laughing, where they can behold us whispering, holding hands. How have Andrew and Dickie aged in place here, in this care space?

Neil Henderson, the late Reygan Finn, Jamil Khan, and Linda Mkhize have all pioneered research on the experiences of aging LGBTQ+ people in South Africa, arguing in general that the present ecosystem of old age homes favors and caters to white women or white gay men.[7] Based on what we've seen so far, I don't disagree.

One of these research articles, by Henderson and Khan, is titled "'I Will Die If I Go into an Old Age Home,'" based on a quote from "Cindy," an older transgender coloured woman who lived outside of Cape Town.[8] In another of their articles, two interviewees, Patricia and Carmen, an older lesbian "mixed race" couple, both political and feminist activists, stated that they feared they would be separated from each other in a place like Grace and surmised that home-based care and or assistance from their children would be preferable.[9] None of the people they interviewed actually lived in an old age home, but most of them recoiled at the possibility.

Maybe Andrew and Dickie didn't try to cultivate a queerer place to age, an Elsewhere or Otherwise place, maybe, in solidarity or community with their aging lesbian, bisexual, and trans brethren of color.

Maybe such an aspired-for community is too hard to achieve, given the prevailing order that codifies intersections of race, class, gender, and sexuality and separates people of color from this mostly white sphere of living, aging, and dying.

Still, I believe we must try to make a place for all of us. One nearer to me, in the United States, is The Pryde. It's soon opening thanks to the activist and advocacy organization LGBTQ Senior Housing, Inc., the only nonprofit in the country dedicated solely to creating and supporting affordable housing for its eponymous communities. They successfully lobbied the City of Boston to rehab-develop a 120-year-old former school in the Hyde Park neighborhood to create a seventy-four-unit rent-restricted complex. Residents can range from earning 100 percent of Area Median Income (shockingly, $103,900 in 2023 for a one-person household) to those who were previously considered homeless.[10] It is the first senior housing space like it in the region, and one of the few anywhere to intersectionally address housing inequities in concrete form.

One night, less than a month after its groundbreaking, The Pryde was vandalized with anti-LGBTQ+ graffiti. Black spray-painted letters read, "there are 2 genders," "die by fire," "die slow."[11]

Maybe, as these researchers argued, older LGBTQ+ adults—Andrew and Dickie, or whomever—are resilient and keep on living despite outright hatred or more muted discrimination. Making community with both their white counterparts who "don't understand them" or the black women and men upon whom they depend to keep their open secret.

~

The cigarette's finished. Andrew looks tired of talking. I don't blame him.

Back to the sitting room, for lunchtime soon. And maybe one last question.

ANDREW

Maybe "to know" is to taste something—to cook, eat, savor, be full.

"We liked cooking, Dickie and me. We went out tons, but we also cooked."

"What was something you cooked for him that he loved?"

"Easy. Roast beef and potatoes."

Like my mom's mom's Sunday special. We used to go once a month or more to her apartment in a subsidized senior housing complex on the West Side. She'd moved there from her village when she retired. She led me off to school after Mom and Dad had already left to work in the morning to teach; or to football practice. The carrots were chunky, inch-plus-long cuts, the potatoes softened, stained chestnut brown in the hours-long simmer.

She bought meats in bulk at Aldi the day her Social Security check cashed. She froze the rest.

As we walk into the sitting room, there's a flash of color on the TV: news coverage about Pride. What's on doesn't look that different from the events I've been to. White men, lithe to muscular, under the snaking arc of a feather boa. Emotions raw, screams of joy, whoops.

Everyone's backs are to us, the permed heads watching, or gazing somewhere else, indifferent to what's on the screen.

"*Gah!*"

Someone pinches my love handles, three or four fingers plucking at my own plaid tucked-in button-up shirt, where the skin and fat lie over the hip bone.

"You need to put some meat on those bones," he says to me, hazel eyes smiling.

Maybe to know *is* to touch. Or to dance.

We take the few extra steps to Annemarie the secretary's office. Andrew does the phones in there sometimes when staff are in meetings, an on-call, in-house answering service.

Bruce is there too. He does the residents' accounts part time and other odd jobs at Grace.

"Andrew, we know on the weekends you're the DJ," Bruce bellows. "He plays that 'oontz-oontz-oontz' music for the tannies." He's thrusting front to back; the office swivel chair's about to explode from under Bruce's bouncing rugby player-thighs.

Annemarie is crying-laughing. Me too.

Andrew's laughing so hard that when the phone rings he barely stops to answer it—"*Grace ouetehuis, goeie dag*" (Grace old age home, good day).

I wonder if Annemarie's ever heard that Ibiza-style 2010s techno music before, what I first think of for the oontz-oontz onomatopoeia, or the deeper dancefloor archives of black and gay house and club music where it was born.[12]

"My jams," says Bruce, "I was born 1982."

"I was married that year!" Annemarie says.

Andrew hangs up the phone.

He's stopped laughing, his mouth still moving,

He doesn't say anything.

Diversity

Angel's back from the funeral, just in time for the next meeting:

Diversity training.

"It was heartsore," she says, settling back in her office throne, fleece sliding off. "Lots of people at the hall. He was Jehovah's, so it's quick, just onto the family things then to his sister's. The kids came from Pretoria. His wife's still down in the cottage here but is going back to Pretoria with the son for a while. They'll probably sell."

Her smoky eyeshadowed lids rise and fall. It was a cremation with AVBOB, an established franchise. Their ads run on TV between the evening soap operas, and in the afternoon to touch those unemployed during the day. They often feature a black auntie waxing grateful for policy coverage.

"I don't know, though," she adds. "They just gave out bottles of plain water. At Pat's funeral there was flavored sparkling. We went with a family parlor that's based in town."

The diversity training officially started two minutes ago. It's a livestream on YouTube. We are one of the seven participants watching online. I think I can count almost thirty people, mostly white-hairs, in the main room, which is also somewhere in Pretoria—some conference venue, not the mother office.

It's chaos.

Angel, Annemarie, and Bruce are struggling to hear the message. The sound's way too quiet. Like Joan and Jane's hearing aids dilemma, we can't quite make much out of anything.

We turn up the volume on the YouTube channel, that little loudspeaker icon—nope.

We turn up the volume on the desktop screen, same icon—nope.

We look for some volume knob to turn on the plastic casing of the desktop—nope.

Annemarie comes back from the storage closet with an oblong speaker, a bird's nest of cables, and a microphone. I'm suddenly missing pre-COVID-era karaoke

DIVERSITY 63

nights at Shanghai Moon back home. She holds the mic up to the desktop screen—a 2D interview of sorts—waves it around a bit, to amplify the little sound we hear. I don't think it's plugged in anywhere.

We try Angel's laptop next. Grace's Wi-Fi doesn't connect to it for some reason. I brought my laptop too, but it doesn't connect either. It does connect to their phones—"Let's try it there." The ladies open Google Chrome on their Huaweis. I look at the URL on the desktop and type it into their phones' browsers.

Loading,

Return to homepage,

And soundlessness—nope.

Thank God in the meantime Bruce went down to the cottages and borrowed someone's external speakers. Plugged into the desktop, the diversity training message starts to come across.

I hope.

Thank God too for "all protocol observed," meaning that the training's keynote speaker hasn't even begun, now ten minutes after the start time. There are lots of other introductions and rituals to get through—the higher-ups at the mother office, random business matters, tea belatedly set up in the conference room, a prayer.

The first speaker is Dr. Melissa Steyn from Wits University. Her titles include Professor and South African National Research Chair in Critical Diversity Studies. I've met some of her students on the campus where I've worked.

"Oh, so you know her already," says Angel.

"Not personally," I say. We have mutual friends and colleagues.

Steyn is a powerhouse. (She has a Wikipedia page.) PhD in psychology, and her master's thesis became the path-breaking and award-winning book *Whiteness Just Isn't What It Used to Be: White Identity in a Changing South Africa*.[1] She's an expert in critical whiteness studies and originated the field of critical diversity studies in this country, also founding an international scholarly journal by the same name published by a progressivist press.

According to the Wits website, her program chairship interrogates the "sometimes subtle, yet systemic and pervasive underdevelopment and even exclusion of those groupings historically marginalised in almost all spheres of economic activity, but notably in key areas of knowledge innovation." The program's research addresses "these social dynamics, unpacking the ways in which powerful systems of sense making shape subjectivities that are invested in retaining forms of organisation that are dominated by, centred on, and identified with, their interests. These hegemonic systems, such as whiteness, hegemonic masculinities, able-bodiedness, heteronormativity, etcetera, intersect and co-construct each other. The implication is that unless an approach that addresses the root dynamics of how power operates upon difference is grasped and applied, little progress will be made towards creating environments that advance all our talents and are open to receiving all our contributions."[2]

"This must all be very basic to you," says Angel.

Not really. I always thought I was better at painting a picture with words—describing what was said and done—than I was at talking about theory. Still, I'm sure we'll learn something critical, something that might get us closer to that Elsewhere I mentioned at the start of this road trip—to freedom.

Dr. Steyn begins with a list of keywords on a slide set, concepts to help us unpack forms of "normative structuring": heteropatriarchy (I don't see the cis- prefix), capit(abl)ism (I've never seen this one before—I like it, makes total sense here), postcolonialism, nationalism, militarism—forces that create difference among us and criteria for what those in power deem to be normal or abnormal.

"I would like the audience to tell me about forms of difference they see around them at work or in their community," she invites.

As far as we can hear, audience members in the room offer "gender," "man-woman," and "ethnicity."

"Good," she says encouragingly, and further explains that sexuality and gender are often problematically construed as binaristic phenomena and originate in Western colonial modernity.

The next few slides have far fewer words. Dark archival images pervade the screen—violence, torture, black silhouettes of human beings with chains around their necks, wrists, and ankles, the pictures of Louis XIV's favorite artist Charles Le Brun, whose seventeenth-century series of naturalistic portraits morphed each figure's anatomical details to depict hybrid human-animal creatures and illustrate a belief that debased personality traits could be read from facial form. (It was called physiognomy.) Dr. Steyn explains that modern Europeans also long believed that non-European peoples were animalistic, subhuman.

"We're all animals," laughs Bruce.

Angel sighs, "That's slavery."

I'm getting anxious. I wonder if they believe Dr. Steyn is talking like she came from the moon, speaking a language that's only partially understandable. I believe she's being professional and professorial. That's her role, but it makes me anxious because I wonder if they believe I'm an unintelligible moon-person too.

She's probably given this kind of talk to hundreds of other audiences who've been a lot less gracious.

I wonder if there's a gap in understanding capit(abl)ism at the conceptual level and figuring out how to diminish its force in an old age home, where Angel or Bruce come to see their own actions and ways of speaking as enslaving, ageist, sexist, or racist. And to then change.

(Good. Let them figure it out. If they do.)

Bruce is messaging his wife about picking up the kids after school. Angel rummages in a filing cabinet.

Next on the slide set is a map of the world's nation-states that shows the extent of European colonization. Nearly the whole world is an oceanic cyan blue—the British.

DIVERSITY

Last is a picture of the skeletal remains of a nineteenth-century woman who lived somewhere in what is today China. It focuses on the feet, broken and blunted, shaped into a diminished size from years of binding. My forensics colleagues might issue trigger warnings before sharing images of human remains like this, but maybe it's not the instructional practice here. Getting desensitized *or* sensitized to such violence is painful.

Helping the learning process, I suggest to my officemates that this gendered form of differentiation included men believing that women had to be petite.

"You know I believe that!" says Angel. "I've probably gained twenty-five kilos (fifty-five pounds) since starting to work here with all the presents and goods that people donate to us!" She adds, exasperatedly, "Men!"

We're sharing a bag of *droëwors* she found in the filing cabinet—dried thin sausage snack sticks made from springbok, a kind of antelope, and seasoned with coriander—homemade. A married couple from town shot the bok and made it themselves. We're also munching on a bag of rusks, and each of us has a cup of instant coffee and a water bottle with Grace's logo on it, like each of the residents receives to stay hydrated—helps with their skin and digestion, says Marina.

Dr. Steyn continues about how some forms of difference are not yet culturally elaborated as negative, as something to be controlled or policed, like green eye color.

Bruce leaves to answer a call from a bank about a resident's monthly debits. Angel quickly answers a call herself—the vet, about a test result for Sparky, her Jack Russell terrier.

"He was throwing up a lot last week," she whispers, "just a virus."

I explain what Dr. Steyn said about eye color, that in the past, for lots of reasons, skin color became the axis of difference used to discriminate and subjugate others.

Angel says she understands. "This is why the blacks hate us."

Now for Q & A.

Dr. Steyn gets one from a higher-up at the mother office, more a comment than a question. "Today, South Africa is not acting on the gift it was given," he declares through the desktop speakers, "the gift of a chance to change itself. We haven't changed. We can teach children to believe things otherwise, that we do not need to fear others."

"Yes," Angel echoes. "A child can grow up learning to hate blacks, but it's the parents who teach their children that."

They could learn it from them, and from cues in society and culture generally, I say.

"But then what about our culture? They always focus on them and not us."

I'm not sure if she means black people always focus on themselves, or if diversity consultants always focus on the suffering of people of color and historical redress.

"Well," I say, not so delicately, "it's more often the case that black people find themselves on white people's grounds and are forced to adapt to a lot of unspoken rules. Some are rude or really disrespectful, or worse. In America, at least. Maybe here it would be something like Mama Zulu moving in and finding that most of the residents speak Afrikaans, so she's forced to adjust."

"Ja, neh" she agrees.

Dr. Steyn gives us breaktime.

Angel calls the pharmacy about Sparky.

~

In the hall, Precious is braiding tannie Little Marie's hair and talking to Gugu, her older colleague, about a home improvement project.

"A sliding door would be nice," Precious opines.

"With an outdoor patio, with tiles. A dream house," says Gugu. "It's more affordable at Cashbuild."

"I saw the prices at the Bushbuckridge store," Precious agrees. "They are."

Gugu shows me her phone's screen image of her three adult children posing in front of an already fine-looking house. It's sunny.

"Born 1984, 1994, and 1997."

"That's quite the spread!" I admire.

"The first one's my birthday twin," Precious laughingly tells us—both born in 1984.

"The first- and last-born are very different, hey," Gugu says.

"You mean in how they see the world? How they behave?" I ask—two "born-free," after apartheid, the other well before. The 1980s were war-torn years, grievable, painful. In the 1990s, people were still grieving, beholding, and making the new postapartheid world in real time.

Gugu says there are *major* differences but doesn't elaborate more than, "The born-frees are all doing drugs," she asserts. "They don't listen!" Young people making noise and bad decisions, apparently. It's a familiar criticism and goes both ways, like Andrew said—the young ones disrespectful and out of control, the old ones who are stuck in the past and must get out of the way to relinquish control.

Precious pivots to other news, another generational horror (and another trigger warning for you). She reads us a story from her phone about a child being found in a vegetable garden, killed and buried there by someone from the neighborhood.

Literary scholar Pumla Gqola calls this kind of storytelling a South African nightmare.[3]

"What should be the punishment for that?" Gugu demands an answer.

"The death penalty," Precious hammers, "but that's no longer the law." It was abolished in the new constitution in 1995, I remember.

"Do you think six to seven or thirty-five years is enough of a sentence for a person who abuses a child?" Gugu demands again. "When they get out, they'll just do it again."

DIVERSITY

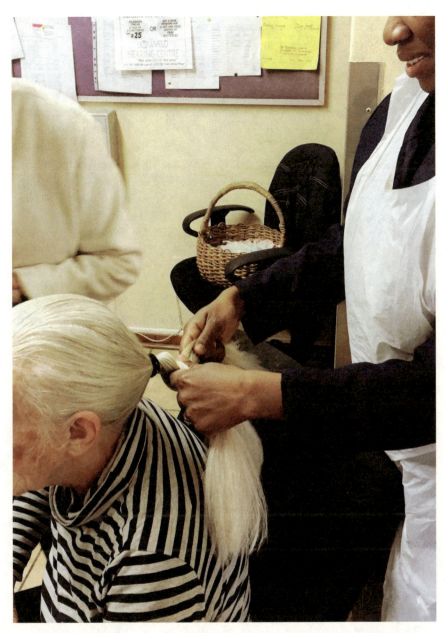

braid

I say the "penalty" shouldn't be legal. It opens the door to discrimination. In the United States, people of color and poorer, less educated people are more likely to be sentenced to death than others, and those whose victims were white. Some of these points were considered in the abolition of the penalty here too.[4] "Something being legal does not make it right, like most of apartheid's laws."

Gugu tsks. Precious just smiles and gets us into another story, partially about the United States. And more tech chaos.

Pretty, the security guard down front, is getting married. She just asked Angel for time off. She has an adoptive mother, Debbie, from the United States. Pretty grew up without parents and Debbie sponsored her through World Vision, a humanitarian program, paying for her school fees and nursing degree. Pretty asked Precious to download PayPal on her phone so Debbie could send her money for the dress and a gift.

Somehow Precious is connected to Grace's Wi-Fi. Angel definitely doesn't give that out freely to staff. None of the residents have Wi-Fi enabled phones anyway.

I don't know where to download the app on her Android. We use the browser to try to make an account, but we need someone's bank details.

Pretty's or Precious's? Do you know the entire account number? Do we need the bank's branch code? But how will Precious then get the money to her?

Loading.

The website asks us to make a password.

Letters, a number, a sign.

Return—it brings us back to make another password, back to where we started.

Letters, a number, a sign.

Reloading.

Return.

And so on.

~

Back to Angel's office and diversity training: part two.

A white woman who formerly worked at IBM runs a session about design thinking. She splits up the audience by age and rank—management, staff, volunteers, ages eighteen to forty-five and ages forty-five and above—and puts them into pairs.

"Looks like it's just you and me," says Angel.

And me to her: "Wouldn't have it any other way!"

The prompt—name your challenges, needs, and pain points. We use pink and white Post-its.

"Learn about each other from what we shared," we hear from the computer.

"What I do is lonely," I confess. "I need to call on my colleagues who do this kind of work, check in with them. It helps me see that what I do matters. I miss Charlie. Mom, Dad."

"Dog food is expensive. They eat a lot," Angel notes. "Without Pat, I'm the one to get up and let them out before work. Take them out, bring them in, open the gate, drive out, lock it again—keep it safe."

"They're back." Bruce steps in to relay the message. "The land grab."

DIVERSITY

Training's over. Angel and Annemarie become wild: "What do they want to steal from us now?" and "They will never stop!"

Angel dials her new CEO who's in the session—no answer—then their attorney.

Bruce spins out some details in Afrikaans: Plaatjieville, a nearby area of macadamia and citrus farms, Grandpa Malopa again, some harsh-sounding words. "Just hang around here, you'll get more action than you were looking for," he laughs.

"Let's go," she says.

Angel drives a long white sedan.

Motoring down to security, we're stopped next to the field of scrub grass and its gravesite as the gate slides open. The wooden stakes, like sentinels, barely cast a shadow in the midday sun.

"Pretty, it's war," she pipes, "and if they get to the gate, don't let them in. If they come with fire, just let it burn and run up here."

Pretty looks calmly and lets us out.

I can't imagine a band of whomever coming with torches to light up an old age home and grab anything.

(Maybe I'm not that imaginative. Or I'm naive.)

"It's the same people who made the grab at us before, Casey, Oupa Malopa and them. They said this land was theirs. That Grace must fall."

Not this time, actually. The call Bruce told us about involved the same group of Grandpa Malopa and crew, yes, but was about a different claim they'd lodged concerning two white-owned farms near Plaatjieville. One of the farmers knows Bruce and the story of their earlier attempted "grab" on Grace. The farmer just called Bruce for some initial advice. Still, Angel's spooked by it all.

Calling it a "land grab" is overkill. It's a claim, in the legal sense, made by Malopa as primary claimant, through the Land Claims Court, a postapartheid innovation for land restitution. It's a government body that tries to settle disputes arising from the country's land reform policy initiatives birthed just after apartheid ended—to mediate claims of who belongs where and owns what, who has right to tenure, to air how land was swindled away from occupants by aggressive or unfounded means, for people who found themselves living on land that whites then later claimed for their own.

Land reform can work on paper, argues lawyer and scholar Tembeka Ngcukaitobi.[5] But like the NHI, it's part of a complex, underresourced bureaucracy often stymied by anxieties, white and black, economic and political. Director of the Institute for Poverty, Land, and Agrarian Studies, Andries du Toit, argues that today "land" and its claims symbolize way more than the material value of the ground beneath one's feet. It symbolizes attachment, rights, and rites to belong, especially for rural black communities who've been denied.[6] For communities and families like Grandpa Malopa's.

I wonder, where do the dead beneath Grace's yard belong? Should they be reinterred where their descendants now live, long after being torn from their own? Should they remain here at Grace, among these older adults—the nearly departed?

I wonder whether the dead beneath us will be the first these tannies meet once they get to the other side.

One kilometer down the road is the attorney's office in a Dutch colonial-style building with dovecotes. Inside, a middle-aged white woman comes from a back room to relieve a young black woman at the front desk.

"Danielle here used to work with me at the bank," says Angel.

The two kiss.

Danielle mourns, "They are back every couple of years."

"If they want the fire, we will give it to them," Angel retorts.

With some sensitivity in her voice, Danielle explains: "Where the claimants live now is too far from town, so they say. So they complain, and making the grab is their idea of a solution."

I mean, I know the reason they live too far from the town—forced removals to racially segregate the town itself. "It will be easier to get to work, schools, and shopping," I add.

"This is not coming back to you," Danielle assures Angel. "Yours is a separate case."

Couldn't they come together, the current owners, the white farmers, the claimants? Like leasing to them for eventual ownership, or buy-backs at submarket rates? Something mutual?

I can tell the two women feel sorry for me ("He just doesn't get it.") To them, my ignorance is excusable not being from here, even though where I am from, the same matters also never die.

Angel ends, "It just ends up going nowhere. We've tried."

I can feel a shred of the sausage stuck between my molars—the hunted bok.

Reloading.

Return.

And so on.

Bethal

"We're getting an ice cream truck!"—the hook for Angel's big announcement at the nurse's station. If her double-decker bus didn't work out, we're still going to find the older adults another set of wheels.

"It's part of the Care Buddies, a new program we want to do, so make sure to get on board," she pleads, waving another large three-ring binder with the details. "We need to get out of doing ordinary things here."

"What does that mean to be a Care Buddy, Ma'am?" someone asks.

"That means actually *talking* with the old people. Getting to know them more."

"Being a Care Buddy means being a special partner for the clients to talk to, go walk with, sit with when we do special things like this truck. Or go swim in the dam," adds Noeline.

"Macadamia takes their old people on a picnic to the dam once a week," scoffs Angel.

Noeline clarifies the side point: "I know many of you can't swim, but we'll fix that. We must learn. Water exercise is good for the old people with poor joints. And if your own child is drowning in the river, you must be able to save them, so it is about you, too. We'll throw you in, but you'll live once you learn!"

Angel resets to the main point: "Part of our job is to care for the old people with a capital 'C,' to help them feel like children again. They get bored of ordinary things in here and it's what we must work against. I know you also feel bored sometimes. But talking to these people nicely is fun. You learn all about them."

I'm finding this out myself. There is an element of "fun," or pleasure in the awe or shock of hearing stories of peoples' lives, and that time itself here feels, well, not "boring," but somehow different—repeating itself, or in suspension—outside of ordinary time.

"Walk this mile with me," says Noeline. "We can't keep going along like the pace of a donkey. Leisure is important and keeps us lively, but so is ethics. Don't be going and telling *everything* you hear to others. Gossip is dangerous. But," she says, pausing, "as you get to know them more, you might hear things you *must* tell us. Say if

Eunice's daughter comes and you see her give her 1,000 rand ($86), you can't keep quiet. If it gets stolen, or they lose it, we are not responsible.

Large money and valuables go in the safe in the office"—security measures.

Angel whips out a clipboard. "So, who will be your confidant?"

The smocked and hairnetted women circle around the sign-up.

"Who's your favorite?" I ask among the crowd.

Goodness chimes in, "Louw! He shares it all with me. We were both police officers once. Or Yvonne, she was too, and a prayer warrior!"

"We're not supposed to choose the favorites," says Bethal, the one man among them.

Precious is next to sign up. She looks at Bethal, and writes her name next to Barra, the former psychologist and opera singer.

"'Beyoncé's mine," she says.

"Bitch," he snickers, referring to Precious.

"This's Bethal," she chides. "He's been here since October. He does the men because they feel ashamed if we women help them. He's like you, Casey."

Face flush—I think I know how. I pretend I'm still giggling about "Beyoncé/ bitch."

"And you would laugh if a fly flew by!" he snaps to her, and to me, "Come. Help me."

He twirls us away from the crowd after signing up for Eunice. Back to unboxing nappies (diapers) in the supply closet. We go in together and shut the door with its skeleton keyhole. In here, a calendar from 2014, a fire extinguisher, boxes and boxes of adult nappies. A wide crack in the tile beneath the door connects us in the closet to the outside hall.

"I'm just back to work from town. Yesterday I was in Pretoria, at the doctor. For the disorder."

"Welcome back," I offer.

Disorder—what's the first thing you'd say if that's the first thing someone said to you about themselves? My own gut, my conscience maybe, goes with "honor it," usually, by asking them more, hearing some truth that clearly must be told— maybe like Andrew's "Nobody knows about us"—something that will explode if it doesn't get out.

It's tough still. I've had friends who want to talk about their illnesses. A lot. It's some people's go-to lead-in, to start any conversation by talking about their suffering or what ails them. It's their truth and testament to living with it, as well as bad aspects of our health care system. Others prefer to hide suffering—their own or others. Others prefer optimism—they also find it's the only way to go on living.

"Are you from around here?" I muster instead.

"I was born at Kabokweni at Themba Hospital."

"That's where they take some of the old people here, I've heard."

"It's true," he says, "and they say old people are like children sometimes too!"

Like the waiting room before, the hospital is a portal, to pass through life's ends and its beginnings, whoever you are.

He's got a large metal pair of scissors; the black paint is chipped around the finger-hole-grips. Almost surgically, he uses one blade to pierce the tape holding together two flaps of a cardboard box packed with nappies.

"But," he adds, cutting methodically, "I grew up in Mahushu."

It's a town known by nonlocals as the way to get to the Numbi border gate, one of the bigger entries to Kruger Park. According to one of the few written descriptions of the township I've read, "Access to the road, rather than public gathering spaces, frequently defines daily life in the community in addition to giving Mahushu its characteristic strip shape that hugs the road . . . Taxis run between the townships along road to the commercial and majority white town of Hazyview, as well as the game reserves and upscale lodges, who employ township residents (largely siSwati speakers) for labor seen and unseen in the international tourism the area receives."[1]

"Mahushu. It was . . ." I begin to ask.

". . . a bit challenging. The life I lived."

First, I think poverty. I hope there was joy. "What did you love to do as a child?"

"Playing, reading, writing stories."

"That sounds fun!" I say, stupidly eager. "Like?"

Flatly: "Games."

Clearly, this is not what he's interested in telling me. This isn't a game.

"Tennis, pushing cars, those bricks wrapped with wire and the bottle-cap wheels, because we didn't have toy cars."

Joy, yes, and the poverty, I guess.

"Mostly with the girls. The males I played with were family. I am the last-born. We were eight children by my mother and father, but one passed away."

"What do you remember most about your teenage years?"

For him, this is where time begins: "It was then I had this problem I was fearing. It wasn't easy for me."

He's not hesitating but still trepidatious. I know he *has* to say something about the "disorder," to me, maybe, or to anyone else, as Precious says, who's somehow "like you."

"Because when I was like thirteen or fourteen, I started developing breasts."

Puberty or gynecomastia, I wonder, letting the story unfold.

Further cutting the box's tape, each slice paced to his words: "I asked myself, 'Why?' You know how teenagers are, saying, 'He's a boy but he's got breasts,' teasing. That's why I think I had a bit of stress, those challenges."

"Were there others like you in Mahushu?"

There weren't.

"I don't know. I was confused. When I asked my mother at first she didn't want to talk about it. I kept complaining. I had to. I kept asking, 'Why, mother?' and 'Why are they teasing me?' Then, I stopped going out. The only time I was going out was to go to school, then come back and stay in the house. At that point, my father said, 'He should get help.'"

What did Mom know, or what did Dad not know?

"We went to the clinic first. That's our procedure"—the order of things, triage—"first the clinic, then the hospital with the referral. We went to Themba, and from there Pretoria. I was eighteen then."

"What was in Pretoria?" I think I already partly know—more resources, more specialists, more acceptance of those who are somehow "like us" in the city.

"A psychologist, tests. They wanted to know what happened to me when I was young. I knew then that my mother knew something."

We're done taking out the nappies from the first box. He hands me the paint-chipped scissors to open the next one.

"She said that when I was born, she saw I had a problem. When we came home from the hospital, it was difficult for me to urinate. She took me back, and they did some operation. They talked about something like a womb, and how it was removed. I was a baby at that time."

"Bethal," I whisper.

"I've always had a scar, but I did not know what for. When I asked about it, she would talk about something else. She never wanted to talk about it."

"Because?"

"Because she didn't want to hurt my feelings. I was too young, she said. I was old enough then. It was the first time I had an understanding of what was going on."

Finally, a light.

"At first I was scared. But then I said, 'No, Bethal.' I said, to myself, 'This is how God created you, that you must love yourself and be proud, no matter what people say.'"

Imago dei, however it is that we are human, we are made in and of the image of God—a quick definition of this theological idea. I'm almost breathless, but say, "What you've faced . . ."

He knows.

"The psychologist helped because we don't have this information at Mahushu or Themba. Like here in practicals, or in school, we learn things. They explained things to me: chromosomes, that I was born with XX, that I can take hormones. They asked me too if I wanted to change my gender."

"Did you?"

Flatly again: "No."

"Why?"

"Because. I wanted to live like I was. The way I am, like I said. The way God created me."

Still almost breathless, "Bethal, it is awesome."

"You think so?" He looks at me in earnest. He knows his power, to do the two-fold, to string out one's curiosity and to enlighten.

It *is* awesome—to self-affirm an exceptional life as divinely normal despite "disorder." To come through the fire. It *is*—to decide to share it all in this moment, and that it should or can be known by you and me, others, those who take this tour.

"They gave me a choice to choose what I wanted for myself. And having that choice felt good."

"But she waited, held off telling you for so long," I counter, "You could've known before."

"I know, but I came to see it in another way—a woman who was trying to protect her son. My father, he might have known, or was covering up that he didn't. I do think that sometimes. But if he did, it was because he wanted to protect me too."

"Are they still with us?"

"Yes, they're in their sixties now, almost seventies."

"Do you think they are 'old'?" I ask, slightly stressing the adjective. We could say *khulu* instead—older, but also greater, wiser. Honorable.

"They are, but not so much like the people here"—at Grace. "They are still strong. They farm vegetables outside of town—cabbages, tomatoes, spinach. If anything, they are struggling with this economy. But even in difficult times, they stand together. They are *the* example of how a couple should be. For raising a child like me."

"And that was difficult?" Simply existing as who we are, in God's image or others, should never make our lives difficult or anyone else's.

"Yes. Because in the olden days when they grew up, such things were not . . . known. And they had to face it."

"Did you feel like a different person afterward?"

"Not really," he says, firmly stacking one packaged undergarment after another, higher and higher, "I saw myself as the same, it was just that I knew myself better. But that was still the most scary time of my life."

We stop stacking before the top two shelves, where an at-home spa-style footbath unit sits unused. No one is tall enough to reach up there anyway.

"But why?"

"I believed I would die"—the real heart of the problem—"the breast reduction. The surgery was also in Pretoria, the same year we went and learned everything. We planned with the doctor, and I said yes to it, but we didn't know what would happen. Mostly, I remember my mother. I remember . . . I saw her crying. She was scared. And I was scared. On TV I heard that some who had it . . ."

His words repeat and unspool,

". . . who had it. And died. I thought that would happen to me."

A deflating sound, air slowly releasing from a package on the shelf is the only sound besides us breathing.

"I was there about two weeks. And then I came back home. I didn't really feel any different. As I came back, I first wondered what people would say when they saw me," he says, sighing.

His head drops sideways to his left shoulder, gazing at me. He's drawn a black ballpoint pen from his scrub shirt pocket, tenderly rubbing its capped end, suspending it in air, near his mouth, as if to take a bite. And then grinning, "But people always find something to say."

I also grin.

"Let's go see Eunice."

Out of the closet, for now, to Room 30.

"Do you think people would change the way they act toward you if they learned all this?"

"There's always gossip, Casey. For me, I say there is no need for that, just talk to me straight! I'm not here to entertain. I've mostly talked about it with everyone, so they know me, and I know myself. I'm fine. The Sisters are fine by it. They know it is a medical thing and that it is my choice."

"And the residents? The old men you help here?"—those who grew up in the "olden days," when these things were supposedly "not known." (They were—just by different names.)

"I think some of them might change the way they behave to me, but some don't. Some know. Did you meet Johann's roommate Johnny? The fat one? He knows because he asked. He said he saw something in me. We talked, and that didn't change us. Who we are together. He understood."

Someone's painted a little green ivy trail along the door frame of room 30.

"For Care Buddies, I was going to put down Barra. We were supposed to choose someone we don't know, not the same ones we talk to every day. But this one, I just cannot pass."

In a well-loved recliner, Eunice snores. She shares a room with Little Little Joanne. Eunice looks like my late Grandma Golomski, my dad's mom. Cropped, still-not-gray hair, big glasses, the smell of cigarette smoke hovering somewhere, like Grandma. Curmudgeonly too. I tell him so.

"She doesn't mind talking," he whispers above the roar, "which I like, and she tells me to 'fok off,' when she likes."

"She's your favorite?"

"For now, I guess. Before, hands down, it was Tony the dentist. He was from Greece. He was my favorite. He was Andrew's roommate for a while, the one after Dickie. We just talked a lot, laughed a lot, when on long walks. He was just, *cool.* And very kind, I can say."

We take her ongoing snoring to be a salutary fok off.

Moving on, we pass into a side room—in it a plastic-sheeted bed, oak chair, a shelf of withered books, mostly romance novels—and through the gated door to the courtyard again. Masks off for now.

"But why are you here, really, Casey?"

I've been getting better at explaining this, I promise.

BETHAL 77

"I hear you," he says. "Old people *are* very important, and we have much to know from them. My grandparents were around when I was small—my mother's side, I didn't know my father's. My grandfather was always away at work, a security company guarding (white people's) farms. My grandmother had a house at Badplaas (eManzana now). She farmed like my mother and father. She was strong. An up and up woman."

"I bet."

"Because of her, my grandfather had the care he needed, after he became blind and bedridden with a catheter. It was terrible. And it made me feel terrible. Bad, I can say, that he couldn't help himself anymore. That he wanted to do for things himself and couldn't."

"It shaped you," I guess aloud, "or helped you to see what it would be like to be a nurse? To care for someone else that way?"

"Wanting to be a nurse, Casey. It came after I went through all the changes I felt. I said to myself, 'What am I doing in my life?' I remember the nurses at Pretoria were good nurses. And I always wanted to help others. So, I guess I wanted to return the favor. I can say it also came from seeing my mother with her mother's brothers and sisters. Some take the pension"—the government's old person grant. "My mother's the eldest, so she takes care of them. She'll take them to the hospital, help them with money and whatever. That's how we were taught. Even when you've got your own children, you must put others first and love them, because in our culture they are very important to you. And," stacking the anthropological factoids, "in our culture, you must take that burden when you're the eldest."

"Boss-lady burden!"

"You can say that!"

The writer Niq Mhlongo asks if it's actually burden or *ubuntu*—the black philosophical concept around here of being humane and showing humanity among the world's other beings—earning a living and siphoning some of little one makes here as a black person to your loved ones, out of heart or "culture."[2] It's probably a burden *and* ubuntu.

Speaking of love again, and flipping through one of the romance novels he's plucked from the shelf—1970s oil-painted cover, a bosomy *boermeisie* (white farm girl) heave-hoed in a pirate's arms:

"Casey. Do you want to get married?"

Again, a face flush: "I do."

Eyes rounding, smiling demurely: "Well, I'm not saying anything. I must start saving up for your wedding."

"And what about you?"

"There is this one guy," he alludes, more enticingly, "but I don't know if we are in a relationship. He's in another town. We met when I went for a referral. He calls me like five times a day," laughing. "I'm not sure what we are. We'll see. Like I said, I'm not here to entertain!"

I'm definitely entertained. Like with Andrew, like anyone we've talked to. How can we not be? This place, named for a Christian virtue, is queer as hell.

"Was this your first job?" I ask. And speaking of Angel's ice cream truck, mine was at a Dairy Queen. Very fitting.

"Yes."

"What about it surprised you?"

Grinning again: "That it was just old people. I mean I knew that before, but then it was clear. It's *just* old people. It was not so strange, but I did think of my grandfather. I saw him in these people"—they're not the same, and yet they are somehow—"and I said to myself, 'I must help these people.'"

"What was toughest?"

"Facing their mental illness, their aggression. But I always stay calm because I learned the theory behind it. We did an Alzheimer's course. When you meet these people every day, you learn that the behavior comes and goes. Sometimes they're aggressive, and you just need to ignore it. If you feel frustrated, just walk away. Because the more you try to answer or fight back, it will get worse."

I think of the agony, mysteriousness, pain depicted in films about Alzheimer's or dementia: *The Notebook, The Savages, The Iron Lady, Still Alice.*

"But it doesn't surprise me anymore. It makes sense. Well, some things do. I remember it was . . . well, I won't say who. I was doing something and went into the dining room. There she was, stripping naked! Just taking off her clothes right there for dinner!"

"And you just said, this has to be . . ." I'm about to say "Alzheimer's."

"A strip club!"

We laugh. Sex and aged bodies are made to be incongruous. They shouldn't go together, we learn, according to the cultural scripts we've mostly absorbed. We're *made* to think it's funny.

"Every day, it seems like I'm learning more about old people. Not about the physical, but about who they are as people."

"What would you do if one of them said something racist to you?"

I ask it knowing that it's what many elder care workers in the United States face on a daily basis. Again, most caregivers, certified nurse assistants and the like, are minorities among their majority-white charges, being women of color or immigrants.[3] It is the case for other countries too, in the Middle East and Southeast Asia. In South Africa, rather, the racial demographic of the paid elder care workforce reflects the racial demographic of the country's majority, rather than the minority they tend to. Elder abuse is not just about elders being abused.[4] They abuse too, whether they know it or not. In the United States, elder care managers sometimes ask staff to let the abusive behavior slide.[5]

And now that I think of it, the films I just mentioned are all about white people living with Alzheimer's. Samuel L. Jackson starred recently in a limited streaming series as a man living with dementia, *The Last Days of Ptolemy Gray,* but there are

BETHAL

far fewer depictions of its effects on black families and relationships, let alone how racism shapes caregiving—whether one gives up on the job or not.

"Do you think old people are more racist in general?"

"They are," he admits, and I assume he means older white people, "but I don't blame them. That is just how they grew up in that time."

"But they can't get away with saying these things, can they? Shouldn't they be punished?" is how I suddenly end up phrasing it.

"How can you punish an old person," he asks laughingly. "You can't!"

"Well, do you think being 'old' is an excuse for bad behavior? I mean, can't people change even if they're old?"

Maybe mildly exasperated: "I don't think so. I mean, they can change if they really want to, I suppose. But most don't, or they won't."

Precious told me another caregiver recently quit because of it, the constant barrage of outright and indirect comments from certain residents. The caregiver wasn't unforgiving, per se, she just didn't need to hear it anymore.

(And maybe you don't need to hear any of this. You've made up your mind already about "old racists.")

"Like I say, I am now used to the same routine, the physical things we do for them. I try to get to know them more and more as people"—I guess the Care Buddies is an easy add on to what some staff already do—"and I do love the work."

"I think they love you here, the manager and Sisters."

"You think so?"

"I do. The way I've heard Noeline and others talk about you. You can tell." Or, maybe that's my impression. And speaking of, Noeline appears behind us in the room.

"My sweets, the delivery just came in. Can you make it fit?"

More donations, "presents"—back to the closet.

"I heard Goodness's mother is in a home like Grace," I let Bethal in on what she told me. "Why do you think black families would put their parents there or in a place like this?"

Thoughtfully: "Maybe it's different where she is. But it's probably because the kids are working. Everyone is so busy. There is no time to look after them and they think the parent will be safe in an old age home."

After all, the home's name means "security."

"Do you think an old age home generally is more of a white people thing?"

"It's not a problem," he says, flipping the question to focus on our immediate surroundings. "The mother office for Grace doesn't mind we're here"—black people in general, he means. "They made a deal with the government so that black people and those who don't have the cash can come here. Grace is reasonable. It's all a good company, I think."

Not a charity, as the new CEO now says, according to Angel.

"I think it is different for them too, for white families. They never come to visit, even when a person dies. That's what I notice."

I'm a bit incredulous at the reported callousness. "Don't you think their children love them?"

Sighing: "Not all of them. Because for us, I wouldn't bring my grandparents here and not see them for like a *whole month*. It doesn't happen. I just think most white people don't take family seriously. They put family last. In here, a parent will be ready to pass on, and maybe the children are in America, like Miss Frikkie's, but they won't come to see them at the end. In our culture, or if I were even in America, I'd have to go home."

I'm wondering about the time lag in this story, and in the person's decline: among the slower, longer period of dying, and then the final hours, the dying moment. The aftermath. Somewhat disbelievingly still, I just say, "Wow, that's sad."

"I agree. For us, even when the undertaker comes around, they won't put your parent in the ground until you get there. In our culture. But here, their kids just say, 'It's fine.' Like you say, it is a 'wow.'"

Back in the closet, only one more box of nappies among other presents from Boxer's, a discount supermarket—toilet paper rolls, baby powder.

"Well, before the undertaker gets them, what do you think most of them want in their lives?"

"Like Sis' Noeline wants for us in the Care Buddies—they want company, to talk to someone. They get depressed, like, they just sit alone in their room, not talking to anyone. It's boring, hey. I would die if I was in here as an old one with them!"

"You would die?" I laugh.

"For real! Maybe it's different somewhere else, like where Goodness's mother stays." By this I guess I think he means that staff and residents have some more common ground, common language. By, for, with black people. Not a postcolonial multicultural hoorah.

His hand with a toilet paper roll in it shakes off the dire prospect: "No, I really can't be doing the same thing everyday wake, eat, sit, sleep. I can support myself by then. Or maybe my brother's kids can take care of me. Or maybe this new boy if he is the one!"

"Now you're talking!"

"I like to talk," he winks.

"I like that you like to talk! We wouldn't learn anything if you didn't!"

~

What we've learned about him, this one man capable of changing perspectives— his parents, his own, ours—about what it means to be someone like him, trans or intersex (and I know I haven't used the word yet; he hasn't), queer, or otherwise.

Some people I know, members of LGBTQ+ communities here, have said "queer" is a word you learn in NGO and human rights workshops. There are few trans men in the public sphere. Noks Simelane, Malik Moyo—others' names grace South Africa's newspapers, making it all the more "normal," moving others toward understanding, acceptance—changing things.

"The big changes in your life happened when you were eighteen, you said."

"I'm almost thirty now," he laughs, "and 'born free,' as they say."

"And thirty years since all of that ended, as they say"—apartheid again. "People like Andrew, Eunice, Sis' Noeline"—whites—"I mean, they're now our elders."

He looks at me blankly.

"I mean, you know, they say we must respect or honor our elders. But they were also part of the problem. Should we still respect them somehow?"

"That is a tough one," he says looking thoughtfully at the remaining box. Some of these nappies will probably get put on Barra, Little Marie, and others.

"It's time we make peace with these people, I think."

This place exudes peacefulness already, it seems, but gentleness, quietude, the garden poinsettias—they're a colorful cover that obscures or silences what's already here: past violence in present scars, ghosts.

"And what about the ones that got us through it? Those aunties and uncles—Zuma, Mandela, Winnie. There were so many promises and dreams. What happened?"

He's faster to answer this time: "The black government failed us."

"Bethal, no."

"Yes. I think it's time they give it back to the whites."

"No!" Part of me believes he's saying this to me *because* I'm white.

Laughing insistently, "Yes!"

"Well, what about the EFF?"—the Economic Freedom Fighters, the anti-capitalist, Pan-Africanist party founded in 2013 as a radical break from the establishment ANC. Their platform includes nationalizing banks and mines and free health care and housing. In 2021, the EFF received 10 percent of the national vote, the ANC 57 percent.

"The EFF is worse! Casey, they will chase you out of this country," he laughs more. (Now I know he's definitely saying this to me because I'm white.)

"The time of Mandela, it was better. Now there's too much corruption. Open TV, it's corruption; on the radio, it's corruption; in the newspaper, it's corruption. It's corruption everywhere!"

What Andrew and Goodness said, what a lot of people here say. I don't disagree, but it's more complicated. Yes, the narrative of "corruption" rearticulates colonial discourses that black political parties cannot "manage," be "efficient," or run things right.[6] And yet, people are also murdered for exposing "corruption" within the illicit political economy inherited from apartheid. I think of Babita Deokoran, former acting chief financial officer of the Department of Health for the Gauteng provincial government which oversees public hospitals in Pretoria and elsewhere. She was gunned down by still-unidentified assailants after dropping her daughter off at school, allegedly for being the whistleblower on an ANC racket involved in illegal procurement of COVID personal protective equipment.[7]

In South Africa, books about "state capture," the name for these now decades-long entrenched practices of governmental or extralegal corruption, are bestsellers beside Afrikaans literature, including romance novels. "It's a middle-class market," one publisher told me.

Suddenly, we're caught. Marina swings open the closet door, surprised that we're still in here, yelping "Oh!" And thank God. Organizing donated care detritus by the hour for an unlivable wage (and my computer's autocorrected from "unlovable" as I type this)—is getting a bit stifling.

"Sis," he greets.

"My love, you can go home early if you want. We'll just make a note about your hours."

His mother had wanted to meet him at a new mall near Mahushu this afternoon to buy a new phone charger. "It's not a good mall," he concedes, "there are too few stores."

Marina seems to have been influenced by Goodness's WhatsApp pictures and information about this morning's protests on the road. The burning tires and staged cinder blocks and boulders to agitate the police or community leaders to do something about the untenable conditions we've inherited.

"Transport is tough these days when the sun rises late and sets early. No one wants to travel in the dark," she adds.

"Sister," Bethal sighs, "it's not about the sun. It's about the light." Sometimes, where he lives, the wires and other materials are pilfered from lamppost lighting on along the roadsides. Sometimes, they just don't work.

"Ack," Marina wrings her hands, and says to me, "It must be safe where you're from," before leaving us.

I won't get into the racist mass shootings.

"Well, if they've failed us for now, Bethal, we can still hope for something new tomorrow. Right? Maybe we need a five-year plan."

"I won't be *here* in five years! But I do want to have my own home. A two-bedroom. And I don't want visitors to feel bored. My late brother's kids can come live with me. We're close. I know I'm not like other guys, Casey, and I'm thankful for that. That I can be a lesson for other people. To show people they mustn't judge others. They don't need to."

"Sage lesson. And what is it that you'd want people to know about this place, Grace"—dying, aging, black and white. "What matters in the end?"

Ponderingly, then definitively: "In life, just do right today. It's like that one song," he says, and then sings his own version of those immortal lyrics by American country music star Garth Brooks:

"If my time on Earth was through,
I'm gone and you must face the world,
Is my love I gave you in the past,

BETHAL   83

Is it gonna last,
If tomorrow never comes."

~

"Casey, I quit."

Bethal and I are eating wraps at a KFC in that mall.

"I went to work at Macadamia"—the ritzier private old age home in town. "We had a black head sister, but she was too rude. She liked money too much. 'You can be gone tomorrow,' she'd say, 'I have lots of people lined up who are waiting for work.' No one liked her."

"With that kind of turnover, you have to spend all your time training people instead of building a team," I suggest. "It's not sustainable."

"I agree. She made me want to quit. But then I found the agency nurse thing. Now I'm down in the cottages when they need me."

In the United States it's called travel nursing: a thirteen-week contract placement at health care facilities around the country via a recruiter with an agency. It was said to have started in the 1970s, when New Orleans' hospitals hired temps to cover Mardi Gras–related surges, the specific length also said to cover another nurse's maternity leave.[8]

Before COVID, there were about fifty thousand travel nurses in the United States, or about 1 percent of the total registered nurse workforce. Between the start of the pandemic and mid-2021, travel nurse positions tripled to nearly 150,000. Travel nurses are younger and more likely to be unmarried and people of color. Mobility, money, and trauma and burnout from treating the sick and dying amid the pandemic are factors for joining. The jobs can pay up to three times the normal staff salary, plus moving, travel, food, and housing stipend.[9] This is also as hospital administrators are not raising wages and fighting the demands of nurses' unions.

Charlie took the same sort of gig. It's flexible, lucrative. Maybe risky.

But not really.

The demand for nurses in general isn't abating. More than half of all nurses in the United States are over the age of fifty. Now, at the same time as aging baby boomers are needing long-term care, many nurses are retiring early or soon to be retiring. Far fewer younger new nurses are replacing them.

"I went to NetCare in Pretoria"—a private hospital—"my first hospital job," he says. "I was nervous! But grateful. They trained me for three days and showed me around. For COVID man, they really dressed you up! Mask, gloves, everything."

I pull my KN95 out of my pocket.

"Yes, it was something like that. After thirteen weeks, I was done. It was doable. Then I came home. Remember Gugu? She gave them my referral. Now when someone in the cottages needs help, I go with the agency. It is easy. I just have one person, not six or seven. The pay is better"—4,500 rand ($263) for every two weeks in the cottages versus inside Grace at 3,750 rand ($220). "One of my client's daughters told me I could make even more going to the UK to care for the old people there."

Angel told me once the agency nurses make too much working in the cottages.

"I had one man down there, a Jehovah's Witness, but he got sick and went to the hospice inside. He passed away."

"I'm sorry."

"Now I'm just waiting for another one."

Safari

Angel's dream's come true: the bus.

Or, a mini-bus, rather. Precious's sister's husband rented it out to Angel for today's recreational trip. On the side, in big blue letters: "Jabula" (Happy).

The passenger manifest lists me, Angel, Andrew, Johann, and Yvonne from inside, and the rest from the cottages: Mr. and Mrs. Malan, Mr. and Mrs. Geldenhuys, Mr. and Mrs. Nels, Mrs. Pretorius. Sexy-man Wayne is the driver.

The requirement of being able to independently transfer oneself in and out of a vehicle—a gerontological "activity of daily living"—means that only less frail residents get the chance to go on these outings. Otherwise, select invites go out to Angel's favorites to make up the final guest list—a lucky thirteen.

Yesterday the kitchen staff packed up brown paper bags of yogurts, apples, raisins, and peanuts. Like I said before, you always need two things on any road trip—a map and snacks. This one might last all day—sunrise to sunset.

I'm in zombie mode. Most didn't mind the pre-sunrise alarm. Some of them would've been up already: the nature of aging and changing sleep cycles.

Mrs. Malan mounts the first mini-bus stair but gracefully turns and bottoms out on the second, sliding down her cane like a firefighter's or dancer's pole.

(I hear from my friend Ieva, a firefighter-anthropologist, that they're actually phasing out such poles because heroes can lose their grip on the way down, or they build single-story fire stations now. I 'm sure dancer's poles aren't going anywhere.)

Mrs. Malan's husband and Angel flank in from both sides—back-up squad to Mrs. Malan's solo that make a few of us cry "whoa" or gasp—to ease her thud.

"Heave, hon!"

Back up and on board. We're not letting one sore ass spoil the trip.

Angel gives me the "please, do it for us, sweetie" look, so I scramble into the farthest back seat, knowing it will be harder for anyone else to get in and out of that spot. I always thought it was the best spot on a South African mini-bus taxi.

86   GOD'S WAITING ROOM

Back there, you won't need to pass other passengers' bills and coins up front when they collect the fare, nor make change for anyone when it's passed back.

The starless, dawn-dark sky envelopes us in stillness. At the gate, Pretty is still on duty, her mobile phone the one light glowing in the guard post. Besides the engine, a few passenger sneezes and sniffles, we don't hear much else or see much from the mini-bus windows. *Unless . . .*

"What's that?"
    Right outside the window. Over the empty patch of scrub grass near the gate, over the ancestral graves claimed by Grandpa Malopa and the community trust. It—something else—is glowing. Hovering,
    Something green,
    Wait, now red-orange, now blue, coiling, like the soul of a fire, its flashpoint oxidizing rare metals in a forge's heat.
    Something undulating like a ridged crocodile's tail,
    Wait, now an elephant's trunk, now an anteater's snout,
    Now nothing.
    Maybe just billowing dust clouds, low to the earth, illuminated by the mini-bus taillight.

~

Pretty lets the gate slide open and close behind us as we leave the fenced-in world of Grace for another, what a lot of people find to be an Eden on earth: Kruger National Park.
    The sun's changing rise and set times, based on our planet's elliptical-seasonal movement, means that the Park's visiting hours change throughout the year. This week, the window is 6:00 A.M. to 6:00 P.M., same as the nurses' shift.
    This month the country celebrates its citizens' diverse heritage. That means they wave some of the Park's entry fees. I realize it doesn't count for me. Whoops. Of course, the apps like Venmo I would use for quick cash sends don't work here. What's developed in North America is meant for that market or Europe, of course, not Africa. Probably related to geopolitics, or some developer's or system engineer's biases about security and corruption issues here.
    In any case, I don't have the cash on me.
    Angel rummages through her purse: "It's on the house, Casey!"
    We cruise for about thirty minutes through the dawning hour along winding roads through Bethal's home, Mahushu. Wayne starts what sounds like the Afrikaners' version of "99 Bottles of Beer on the Wall."
    "Naughty boy!" tickles Angel. She croons us into another about a little chicken and a little flower as we pass the farms—citrus and macadamia orchards—most

SAFARI

advertising the pesticides they use and their on-site bed-and-breakfast lodges to cater to tourists who'd be on their way to paradise.

A zone of leisure, conservation, and labor, Kruger National Park has both a centrifugal pull and expulsive push. In its 1898 creation, the men who worked for Paul Kruger began forcibly removing thousands of black people from these lands—leaving the remains of their homesteads and their buried family members behind—gradually capturing or and fencing in thousands of plants and animals deemed to be "native." Today, Kruger continues to cleave the land into two worlds—a pristine, "wild" world of what things supposedly *used* to look like without (black) people living there versus the modern, postindustrial, peopled one we all live in.

Or it tries to. The fences sometimes fail, animals like lions escape and kill animals like cattle owned by the Park's black neighbors. In turn, those neighbors kill the lions.[1] The Park draws in thousands of workers and millions of tourists each year during its visiting hours.

Already, as we pull into a lot, dozens of other happy buses are unloading passengers like us, reloading them into smaller vehicles that will be less disturbing to the environment inside.

An older black man hawks powder mix cappuccinos for 25 rand (about $1.25) from a pushcart to my fellow travelers, his white age-mates, as we pass through the gate into the wild world to view God's creatures—god-creatures, maybe—from the mediated plane of locked mini-bus windows. A better view than the usual National Geographic on the sitting-room TV.

Mr. Geldenhuys has already finished his snack pack. Between us three in the backseat, Mrs. Geldenhuys passes around a bag of black, white, and magenta licorice Allsorts as the creatures appear:

One nyala, nine waterbuck, nine kudu, another four, then thirty giraffes.

Wayne hollers "camel horse!" every time we see one. (It's a joke—the giraffe's Latin name, *camelopardalis*, sounds like its Afrikaans name, *kameelpeerd*.) Angel groans.

After thirty-one camel horses, I stop counting.

"Wayne, stop for Christ's sake. Let's have a look!" squawks Mrs. Nels. "Happy" the mini-bus stops at a muddy watering hole, the other tour buses crowded there like thirsty beasts. A driver from another alights to photograph an eagle, unmoving and high in a dead tree. I watch, nervously remembering the *Game of Thrones* visual effects editor who was mauled and killed by a lioness the moment she rolled down the car window while touring another game park here.[2]

Brown nubbins surface here and there on the water, molded to massive mounds of unseen, submerged floating flesh—hippos—"sea cows," Wayne hollers.

"Not my favorite," quips Mrs. Geldenhuys. "Look, more like piggies!" she adds, still softly popping Allsorts into her mouth, her gold and pearl bracelet slides gently up and down her thin wrist, lightly sun-spotted brown like a giraffe.

"We had a pig as a child," Mrs. Geldenhuys continues, starting to remember her past. "Named Bernice."

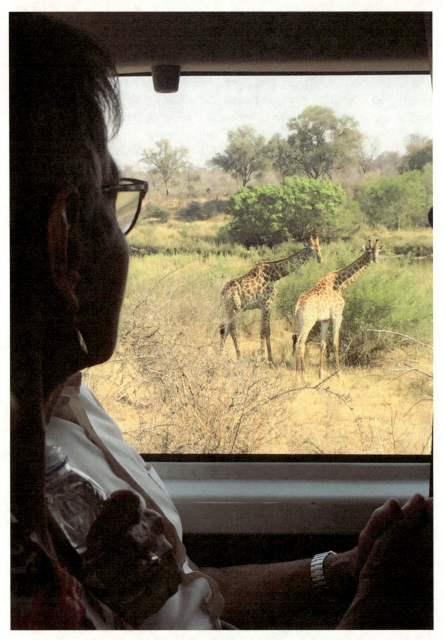
captivity

That was Grandma Golomski's name, I tell her.

"A white one!" she explains further. "She'd sit in the circle with me, my sisters, the neighbor children. We'd drop the little kerchief on her head and run. *Vroteier!*"

"Rotten egg" is the English name of their children's game, a version of duck, duck, goose.

SAFARI

"Fun times," I smile.

"They were. With my granddaughters too. They moved away with my daughter to Johannesburg. No pigs there, of course. She said, 'Mom, come stay with us.' 'Shit, Laura, I've lived here for fifty years,' I told her. 'I don't want to.' I just like to go on with things as they are for now."

Looking outside the window, on the ground, there's plenty of feces strewn about. Wild pigs' too, maybe.

"Don't mind the 'shit,' please," she winks, "it's my favorite word. I played darts for years, for the Free State team even. The girls gave me a set with 'shit' on the tips!"

Suddenly, more gasps—Wayne breaks as a herd of elephants begins to cross the road before us. We all let out ooohs, aaahs, and Mrs. Nels singingly counts, "Two babies, three babies, four babies!" Unbelievably, joyously, we see ten baby elephants pass before us, accompanied by an old paternal guard, a grandfatherly, leathery rock-like god-creature—an ancient one.

Writer Bongani Kona recalls a story by Antonio Tabuchi, about the circle of life from the perspective of an elephant. Kona starts by noting he had just moved back in with his mother in Cape Town because she needed help to make it each morning by 5:00 A.M. to her dialysis appointments. Kona's homecoming marked a full circle, like an elephant, which can sense that another's death is near. A dying elephant picks a companion, big or small, and they walk together until the dying one picks a final resting place. She traces a circle in which the companion may not enter. She transitions, in gratitude to the companion, and the companion returns to the herd.[3]

"Sometimes, we're called on to accompany the one who is dying and we don't know how close they are to that circle we're not allowed to enter and we don't know when we'll be told to turn back," Kona writes, "and because life is circular, someday it will be you and I selecting a companion to travel with us."[4]

We may not know when we will be told to turn back. But I do believe that caregivers, maybe like nurses' aides, domestic workers and others across generations of racialized laborers—people like Bethal or Precious, perhaps—come into a sacred role and knowledge derived from their intimate position along borders like the circle. "Races," castes, life and death—other borders that falsely separate us. Many caregivers come to know when *they* must turn back—not just for the dying, but for themselves.

I also believe there is power in this sacred intimacy, a power that draws together two or more—the dying one, the one who accompanies her, family—to see together that these borders are permeable. To see where each of us stands now as part of the circle, and where we will move next along or across its unending line.

"Stop!" Mrs. Nels squawks again. After the elephants, a troop of monkeys.

The bus reverses so we can gaze. The scene: a small one in repose, lying in the arms of a larger one who strokes its arms. In the briefest moment, it looks like the small one's deceased.

"Can you believe it?" she snaps, "They are running around with their dead babies. A bunch of monkeys!"

Wayne steps on the gas, and the pair jump to life to avoid the tires.

"Shit!" jumps Mrs. Geldenhuys.

"Oooh, oooh," Mrs. Malan grunts like a monkey, rapping the window with her fist.

"They're naughty ones," says Mrs. Nels. Her husband chuckles at the story he knows she's got coming for us. "We loved to camp here," she continues, "the Pretoriouskop spot, eastern side. Once, a baboon got into the caravan! We had biltong and lunch on the table, and it took the whole bag. I just *screamed!* It jumped from there, to there," flicking her own thin wrists higher and higher. "And then, it sat right on the toilet and looked at me like . . ." Her bridge makes the toothy grimace artful, like gleaming Portuguese tile. "This is also why we have bars on our house windows."

"We kept a baboon chained in the yard," Mrs. Geldenhuys adds, "the neighbors rather. It had enough reach that it'd run right up to you when you passed by. Once he ripped my green dress right off me!"

"Naughty boy!" laughs Andrew.

The sun's gone beyond its midday rise. Time for lunch, and the bathroom.

First stop, a campsite that's lush but already overrun with other tour bus groups, luxury-looking ones. Wayne can't find a place to park.

"Shit!" again. Moving on.

Forty kilometers later and wincing from full bladders, we get to another campsite. It's now a searing 32 degrees Celsius (90-plus Fahrenheit). Not so lush, and overrun with school groups of small, small children—preschool even—and their women teacher-guards. Wayne finds a place to park.

The camp visitors still segregate somehow. On the one side of the campsite's café and gift shop, many multigenerational black families cooking out. Thick smoke, steaks and chops, laughter. One the other side, us older whites and the preschool children, two ends of the mortal range, both with snacks in brown paper bags, laughter. Cries and coughs.

Still, a cleansing brings the two sides together in a single queue: the handwashing station. Again, it doesn't matter who you are. You wait.

Angel's gone to rent a grill. More vervet monkeys scamper in and out of the bush, among the picnic tables, looking for dropped snacks, tidbits. Brilliant blue and black birds dart from the fever trees to do the same, squawking like Mrs. Nels. Her husband chuckles again, calling them a derogatory term for people of South Asian descent.

Rolling my eyes, I spoon side-dishes onto everyone's paper plates—potato salad, carrot, pineapple, and raisin salad. Angel's back now and lights issues of the *Sowetan* and *Lowvelder* newspapers she's picked up somewhere, to fire up the rented grill. The men of Grace watch us *braai* with a gendering stare.[5]

"We've moved Frikkie, Little Anne's roommate," Angel tells me, turning the now-oozing *boerewors* sausage. "Doctor Chungu came last week. Noeline thought she'd take a drip"—an IV—"but his recommendation was to just to keep her comfortable for now. If she goes soon, that's two more beds, and we need the open space. Remember you went to Silverdays?"—the poorer old age home in the isolated town. "It is closing this month. Money problems," she sighs. Then, proudly: "They never did things like this there for the old people."

Wayne lays down the finished sausages in crusty beds of rolls, condiments laid out of lime pickle achar and tomato and onion sauce that stains its Tupperware a savory orange.

For dessert, ice cream cups—not from a truck but another older black man, like the cappuccino vendor, like Grandpa Malopa maybe, selling nearby from a pushcart.

Like a tongue depressor, the wooden ice-cream spoon dryly sliding off my tongue feels revolting.

Angel calls the time—homeward bound.

Before that—the restroom. Again, with gendering stares, we queue toward one of two thatched roof buildings with now-fading pink or blue warthogs painted on their plaster walls.

And one last "Shit!" from Mrs. Geldenhuys. Sweating mildly with Mrs. Malan in her arms, she calls me over—"I cannot hold her should she fall. Help her there," she begs.

I aid the cane-using woman to take her final runway walk, the remaining twenty meters through the dusty parking lot, ankles swollen, overfilling her shuffling sandals.

Eating bread, the preschool children go quiet as we pass.

Mrs. Geldenhuys and Mrs. Nels take her inside the restroom to finish the job. No thanks given, just what has to be done. And now I've really got to go too.

After fifteen minutes, we're all aboard, except one: Mr. Malan.

"He has Alzheimer's," Angel whispers to me, unnervingly. "Go check the toilets again. I'll keep looking." And suddenly, I'm sharing her vision of what could happen to the old man if he got lost in the Park.

(Khaki shorts, knee-high socks, bits of his garments torn and shredded, stained blood-red, stuck among the bushes' thorns are all that's left. A black and blue bird darts in, picks one tidbit of fabric, flies off to tuck it into its nest. The aftermath of something ferocious, of violence.)

"Mr. Malan?"

It's dark in the men's restroom. The power's out, of course. I hear nothing, slowly creeping down the line of ten toilet stalls. Outside, I hear Angel calling to him gently in Afrikaans, offering a feminine voice he might hear and respond to—it sounds more like his wife's voice rather than my strange accent.

In the last stall, the door ajar, he's quietly arranging himself by a ray of light from a small window. Outside, for another few minute, we wait until he's done.

The preschool children again go quiet as we pass.

Angel's old people close the windows,

Buckle their seatbelts,

Lock the door.

Goodness

"O,"

Noeline indicates, wiping the counter for the ritual. "O positive. That's Johnny's type. Can you go fetch the man? He won't wheel himself, neh!"

Johnny the veteran stays down in C wing, once part of the South African Army's incursions into then-Southwest Africa, now Namibia, in the 1980s. Maybe he and Wayne fought together. At the end of the hallway of gurneys and cleaning carts is Precious listening to her colleague named for pure virtue, Goodness, speak of more blood and soldiers:

"I heard my own pastor talk about Matthew"—the Gospel, chapter 8, verse 9— "and sis, what he said went straight to my heart. That we are under the power of God, and under us we have soldiers that come and go. They must work for us, but there are challenges to make them do it. But we can conquer through the Holy Spirit. That's me with these soldiers."[1] Thumb turned back to thump her breast: "Inside me, they're strong, and I have hundreds and hundreds now."

During the worst of the AIDS pandemic years, "soldiers" became an accessible euphemism for people here to talk about their white blood cells, or the CD4 count one learns as part of regular screenings.[2] "You need them to be strong. It's easy to check at the clinic," she instructs.

Her sermon's one her colleagues have likely heard before. Many people around here go to church or live a more-or-less normal life with HIV now because they do these screenings.

"Hhayi man, Johnny"—whoops, "oh no, man," in disbelief. Goodness remembers she's supposed to fetch him.

He's waiting for his pick-up at his room's door for the drive to the nurses' station. Our convoy—Precious, Goodness, me—wheels him back to the now-clean desk. Johnny steadies himself by his large hands on the chair's armrests, rising and meeting the rest of us, face-to-face.

Thrust, prick—guided by a laser point, the garnet globule drops on the tab. The women watch the wound, the collective power of medical vision encouraging a successful coordination of red, light, paper.

"It's not always so quiet around here," he huffs, noticing our watch. "Those crazies down there get wild," referring to his room neighbors who live with dementia.

Goodness laughs: "He's the boss down there! He tells them!"

"*Dankie* (Thank you), Captain," salutes Noeline, finishing the test and recording Johnny's glucose reading in the Kardex. "No sugar today, neh," anticipating teatime in an hour or so.

"Let me take him home," clucks Precious, moving into place at the wheelchair's rear, "he's my boyfriend now."

"Bah," Johnny groans.

Goodness asks me to join her on her shift duty—sitting and watching the A wing residents, those living with dementia, the now-mostly-silent, who sit for hours not minding the goings-on around them. Content, maybe, or waiting for something to appear that she and I cannot perceive. She'll bring them to the bathroom, make sure their water bottles are full and that they occasionally rehydrate, spark some stimulation—be their Care Buddy confidant.

We can do all that while talking to each other.

"Casey, what the Sisters need to do is keep me going with my education. I always want to improve. They send some of us to go do nursing"—beyond a caregiver certificate program. "Some went to Susan"—Strijdom, the name of the nursing school attached to another old age home in Pretoria run by one the country's oldest Afrikaner women's organizations.

"How did you know you wanted to become a nurse?"

"Because I didn't want to be in the police anymore! I was on the reserve, actually, for three years. We trained at Hoedspruit. I can shoot when we need to. We learned how to connect and disconnect when we need to clean it," her uniformed arms miming the mechanics of unmaking a gun. Nursing, policing. Both bloody ordeals.

The tense of her statement catches me off guard. Who or what needs to be shot at the old age home? Maybe the land grabbers who might show up at the gate, Angel and Bruce think, an armed nurse taking out community activists in a blaze of glory to save the residents.

(We have legislators in the United States who also want to arm schoolteachers.)

"What did you shoot?" I ask "what," not "who."

"Brown boys we called them, rifles, but I never shot anyone. I quit because the corruption was the problem. They're worse today than back then."

I wonder when was "back then."

"I saw it in what they did about stolen property. You could go to the police to say, "Hey, the criminals stole my TV, the fridge,' whatever, and when they come to your place, they just look around and do nothing. They may have recovered it somewhere and say nothing to you, and when you make the claim or follow-up, they threaten to kill you! I started to say, 'Ha, no, these men are frauds. If you're honest around here, you can die quickly,'" she states.

"Danger zone."

"Ja, so then I decided, maybe I can be good at the nursing thing. I told myself I want to help the helpless people. Nursing is about love and patience, I believe. I wanted to do that for others. The nurses who treated my daughters did too, but there were others I saw who did not, and that inspired me to do it better."

On her phone, she opens an album of photos not originally shot with the phone itself. Here's one where she's one of six in white uniforms—graduation day—the vinyl banner behind them says "Zigna." It was the first black- and woman-owned training center accredited by the Health and Welfare Sector Education and Training Authority in 2000. It's a government accreditor for educational institutions in whatever sector, assuring graduates gain skills that align with postapartheid national development priorities like addressing the critical nursing shortage.

Here's another of her and Janice behind the nursing desk at Grace.

"Your daughters, they needed treatment?"

"Yes. There are three daughters. One is Prayer, she is doing the commission for Old Mutual"—the financial services provider that specializes in term life coverage for the masses—"and before, she was at AVBOB"—again, the funeral provider, for the masses. "My other daughters passed. One when she was eleven."

"Oh, Goodness."

"Cryptococcal. They say there are three types of the meningitis, but I know it was this one. When I took her to Themba"—the township hospital—"it is a seven-day disease. They transported a drip for me from Joburg, and they put us in an isolation room. The drip, I remember, was a sweet, sweet pink. Not watery like a drip can be. It must be covered. The sun must never enter."

"Goodness," I say again, more softly.

"Six drips came, but not the last. On the seventh day, she passed."

"God."

"It did stress me, not knowing why these things happen. But after the police, I went into nursing. I learned that you can get that disease easily when you are positive (HIV). And that when you are stressed this can make you feel worse."

It does—to rot from worry.

"But you heard me say to Precious, I've tested. I know my soldiers. I know how to keep healthy. And that was the best, because I learned a lot about what could happen. Even with this last thing, COVID, we all got the vaccine. And finally, just finally, I made peace with my mind."

The only other people who hear her testimony besides us are three residents—Little Marie, Miss Motsa, and Mama Zulu. Little Marie is scowling in her heart-appliquéd sweater. Mama Zulu is chatting at Miss Motsa. Miss Motsa flops her hand in Mama Zulu's direction.

"Time to drink!" Goodness decides. To the kitchenette sink in the rear of the room for a fill-up, after rounding up the three women's water bottles.

"Here you go, Marie." I offer the scowler a full one.

"No, Afrikaans-only for that one," Goodness corrects me, and to Marie, "*Drink, tannie!*"

96 GOD'S WAITING ROOM

Little Marie winces.

To Miss Motsa, she instructs, "*Vala 'mlomo*" (Open your mouth). She guides the sipper to the blind woman's lips before returning to end the topic of her daughters, and turning to the time when she was their age, a young woman.

"All my daughters are my first husband's—Patrick. We met in high school"— in an area called Bushbuckridge—"I got pregnant with my first one in 1993 and finished school in 1995."

One of the first to graduate in the new era of freedom—not only in South Africa, but the world over, in places like East Germany and the USSR where "communism" and authoritarian regimes also transitioned to democracy. Awestruck, I wonder,

"What was it like then?"

~

Much has been said about what it was like then—for Goodness and others of her generation becoming adults near the end of apartheid, in communities like hers within or near to the "native" reservations turned homelands for black people like KaNgwane, Lebowa, and Gazankulu. In the homelands near Grace at that time, the ANC and other anti-apartheid political movements aimed to recruit the burgeoning youth population to their cause, but most youth turned to address the withering conditions internal to their underdeveloped communities and schools, protesting older politicians' ineffectiveness, corporal punishment by teachers, and school fees. Some young black people formed vigilante-like "crisis committees," and black homeland police tried to counter them. One committee, called the "Comrades," gained huge popularity among students like Goodness. One man, interviewed by anthropologist Isak Niehaus, remembered how prior to joining the Comrades he and his peers roughhoused and played soccer. After, they mobilized the masses[3]—to change their impoverished circumstances,

Wrought by decades of racial capitalist dispossession, political strife among local leaders vying for power, and loss or mutations of ritual practices that once healed and cohered their communities. These circumstances fractured people's capabilities to live well, control their lives, and care about others. Young people and some adults put these fractures at the fore in their quest to change it all—to reclaim dignity, to motivate the masses to create a future Elsewhere or Otherwise they imagined was possible—understanding that they were living amidst forces that were profoundly "evil."

"What it was like then," and what Goodness and her peers did to make this imagined future real, may at first appear surreal.

"Eish, man, those days!" she laughs. The struggle! I'm telling you, there were witches *everywhere*. I was a Comrade, a corporal for the witchfinders. The police fought *us*

GOODNESS   97

if they found out that we insulted the witches! We'd get chased right out of town! If they caught you, they'd take you to the police station, beat you, and bag you! Those big bags for mealie meal (ground maize), you know? They put you in with a cat and threw you in the river. That thing will scratch you to get out until you say, 'No, no, I confess!'"

The cat's out of the bag now, for real. Witchfinders? And "confess to what?"

"Confess that we were out to attack witches. Remember, we Comrades weren't about the ANC or Mandela fighting people like you, Casey"—white ones. "Other people did that fight for us, but we sometimes joined. When the black police who worked for the whites would shoot at us, they'd say, 'We are not shooting you (another black person), we are shooting at the picture of Mandela on your T-shirt!'"—one famous man among many unsung men and women who symbolized the anti-apartheid struggle. "But then, they'd also shoot at us for attacking the witches!"

"And what do you mean, 'witches?'" I ask, even if I think I know what she could mean.

Anthropologists have had a lot to say about the people said to be "witches" in history and all over the world, and the social, economic, or seen and unseen forces witches are said to represent.[4] Two of Goodness's neighbors out in Bushbuckridge were Edith "Kally" Shokane and the late Eliazaar "Jimmy" Mohlale, and, over the years, they've helped anthropologists like Niehaus, human rights activists, and others understand what drives members of their communities to personify evil in one of their own—be they criminals, older adults, or some of the most vulnerable.[5]

One apt definition of a witch is a person who gets socially "excluded" from society or is "othered" to epic, other-than-human proportions[6]—those in power come to believe the person errs too close to the nonhuman, the animal, or the spiritually evil, or acts too strangely or dangerously for the collective good. For this, they must be purified or punished.

On Sundays, Charlie and I used to run across the bridge and brackish Danvers River from Beverly into the ground zero for witches in America—Salem, where colonial white Christian families, some of them enslavers, jailed or executed over two hundred of their own kind in the 1630s. Most of the accused were women, and many were impoverished. Some were at odds with more prosperous accusers. Today, Halloween in Salem is a carnival-like spectacle, with tens of thousands of masked visitors seeking to touch the past and present of the pagan and said-to-be satanic. For these witchfinders, there's always high police presence.

"Casey," taking the pains to say it plainly, "in our culture, if you're a failure, or you're really struggling, you think you are being witched by someone. Or if you do that to someone else, you're a witch. When the Comrades learned someone could be a witch, we went straight to their house to see for ourselves."

"And what did you see?" I don't hesitate to ask.

"You know we are by the Kruger Park, so sometimes you see baboons and monkeys walking the street. But then you might see them go in and out of someone's yard. Again and again. If someone noticed, we could watch in the night to see it. We went door-to-door getting donations from their neighbors. They'd pay and let us pass and search the yard for the animals or things a witch left behind. It's a lot of work, so we need to get paid too!"

"And if you found something?"

"They killed them," she half-smiles.

The heart of the Comrades' "insults" the police investigated.

"Sometimes we just burned their house," she adds. "They'd run away before we got there."

I look away to light reflecting within Mama Zulu's water bottle.

Last week on the road trip, I tell Goodness, I visited a daytime activity center for older adults in Dwaleni—the Rock—that township behind the airport. Like Angel, the manager there Mr. Mabuza told me about their daily operations, goals, and challenges.

After the tour, he showed me a pixelated video clip on his Samsung of a destitute-looking older woman in a shredded jump suit surrounded by police, who are themselves surrounded by dozens of people. He told me that what I was watching was an attack on the older woman, "because they think . . ."

". . . they are also witches"—she finishes my sentence.

I try not to look directly at the older women sitting nearby. Little Marie is snoozing. Mama Zulu's chatter is now more quiet and to herself. Miss Motsa is rolling a ballpoint pen to- and-fro across the table.

"Since then, I learned people can think funny things about someone just because they are old. Isn't it that if you become old, your skin looks different, like in shingles or dryness?" she ponders. "The hair changes and leaves. When you look into the blacks of their eyes, it seems so deep, deep. You start to think, 'Who are you?'"

Who all of us will become.

"They can do funny things too. They might whistle or walk in the night, and if we get up to see what the noise is about, we see the person may be standing there, naked in her yard."

I recall Bethal's aha moment, the episode about the stripper of Grace.

"So we thought they could be a witch"—seemingly because of strange behavior or their appearance—"but it wasn't just the old, old ones. Comrades looked for the very, very bad ones too. The ones who hurt other people. Who are corrupt or steal"—and again now, I wonder if trigger warnings are needed in recounting some tales here—"They'd catch the witch and make them drink petrol. Then, a cigarette goes in the mouth, and someone says, 'Light the switch.'"

"Goodness, God!"

"That's what it was like then," she half-smiles again, "the courts and law do not believe in witches, so we had to fight for ourselves. We were more angry at people who did robberies, rapes, and stealing, ones who poisoned their own husbands and wives for money and things. The Comrades are not around these days. It's always a generational thing. The younger generation wants to fix things fast fast and take matters into their own hands."

The younger generation, like Gugu her coworker complained about, believing they can control at least one small part of the larger world that seemed to be out of control. Niehaus argued that the Comrades "gave powerless individuals"—often young and economically bereft people like themselves—"the necessary public support to accuse neighbors and kin as witches, and although many elderly people felt intimidated by the Comrades, it can be argued that this was a consequence of, rather than a motivating factor for witch-hunting."[7] In this instance, it happened to be one marginalized group dehumanizing another.

When it comes to race, it is often the same case—where many suburban and rural working-class whites come to dehumanize immigrant people of color.[8]

"I can see now that we were killing innocent people sometimes," she notes, "but then again, when we showed them what we found in the yard or told them we saw their baboons, they confessed."

~

To bring her from the past to now, to understand how an older adult can shift in mind from the figure of a witch to a geriatric care recipient, requires another confession—"When you started here at Grace, were you surprised to see that it was only older people?"

"Too much."

"Too much?"

"Too much," she laughs, "I mean, eish, OK, my heart was very, very down. Because I thought about the previous things we did to people like them. And when I started to see them here, physically, it was a heartsore to me."

Again I think of Bethal, or any staff member here, who acquired "theory" about geriatrics, when the "practical" is what you would learn, know, or do already in your everyday interactions with older family and neighbors. Many black South Africans already live in multigenerational households.

"At Grace, I started to understand as I gave my ear to them to listen. Sometimes, we don't. That's why they want to do the Care Buddies. But it *can* be hard to stay at home with an old person if they have dementia and begin to repeat themselves."

I remember reading an article from the 1990s about Xhosa-speaking people's perceptions of people living with dementia. They characterized their repetitive actions as being constantly on "rewind," like a videotape, the more obvious technological metaphor back then.

"It's like they think *you're* the stupid one, that you didn't hear them the first time. Or when you tried to dress them, they put on three clothes at the same time, or none at all. If you have siblings like me, and one visits the parent, the parent may say something like, 'Yoh, no one's fed me, what am I going to eat,' when one of your sisters did so. They're insulted, or think, 'If my father or mother say this, it means he doesn't love me.' Before, we used to call them out if they sounded like they were lying, but now I know it's Alzheimer's and dementia. They've only forgotten what they've done."

The potential for different interpretations about what's happened is great—yesterday becomes more and more like mystery than history.

"But how do you get to the point of hating your older parents for it"—not hating, maybe, but chasing them from the community, or worse, seeing them as a witch—"Do you know what I'm trying to say, Goodness?"

"I know what you are trying to say," she says, seeing I don't get it. "We love and respect the elderly, but a family can turn its back if they don't understand these changes. Remember that if you're a failure who doesn't get married, find a job, or have children, you look for answers as to why, and some go to a *sangoma*."

Sangoma, *inyanga, dingaka*—a healer, someone who's adept in divining answers as to why you experience one or more of the problems she lists. Someone who's learned how to dwell in the shadows where life and death converge, to commune with ancestors—yours or their own. They're sources for understanding your problems as possible generational curses or trauma, or for knowing to whom you must sacrifice or make reparations.[9] To many, healers are mystifying.

"And sometimes they're false prophets," she clarifies. "They'll tell you"—in a gnarled voice—"your grandmother or grandfather is witching you. But"—she pivots to a critical, clinical voice—"some are false and use your information against you. If he asks about the grandparents, and you tell him they've died, then the false ones tell you they're not resting in peace. Or if they are acting strange, it's because they're witches. Not all of them are lying, just some. Some, when they're ready to die, confess saying, 'We were just making money by saying these things.'"

My colleague Erica tells me we still do not know much about "deathbed confessions," empirically at least. Many world religions have it on their books as a must-do before you go. Legally, they can be admissible as evidence in a U.S. court of law. Cathartically is how they tend to work in a Hollywood movie or book for complicated characters who need to get something off their chest in the end.

"And the Comrades never went after a false prophet?"

"I never saw that. If the false one died, I guess we just went to their funeral," she laughs. "Some have the calling and become a sangoma, but others stop doing it after a while and move on. Like Mama Zulu over there."

The resident in the pink knit cap who is still sitting at the table with us squeaks at hearing Goodness say her name, "Yebo, *'nkosatan* (my girl)," directing her gaze to her caregiver.

"Mama Zulu is a sangoma?" I almost shout. Goodness looks at me like I should already know this fact. It's a story for another chapter.

Mama Zulu listens in and Little Marie, awake now, scowl-surveys the room in our general direction as Goodness reiterates, "The spirit of love developed inside of

GOODNESS

me, telling me that we must love people unconditionally. Because old people, all people, deserve to be loved. Even if they are about to die, or the mind is not there, we cannot neglect them. They still have rights."

I'd be keen to hear what a social worker would say about her story so far.

"I am a Christian because my father was a pastor in ZCC," she adds, the Zion Church in Christ, one of the biggest churches in the country, nearly 5 million members and established in the early twentieth century by black African converts and visionaries' encounters with white missionaries from Zion City, Illinois.

"He had many jobs and did much for the people around here," showing me more images on her phone of her father—one of him holding a black-and-white photo of himself from the bygone era, and other photos of the same kind spread on a doilyed table. "He took boys from Bushbuck' to the cities to be cooks in the white people's homes. The Smiths, they were. He worked in factories in Germiston and was a hospital custodian. Then he became a police officer."

Like father, like daughter.

Her finger daubs to another phone photo album to open another picture of her father, Calson, late 1970s, early 1980s, I guess—the late apartheid years. His green uniform says "Department of Agriculture and Environment," a nearby car's license plate beginning with "GH"—Gazankulu homeland, for people of "Shangaan ethnicity," as one's passbook or ID would say.

"He was in the police that protected nature and the Park (Kruger). The people around here got firewood from the Park or water, find honey, shoot birds or hunt animals that the whites say are protected. Most times he didn't 'arrest' the ones in the community. If he found them doing something wrong, he just said, 'Sorry'"—gotcha—"and tried to encourage them to be better. But then his commander warned him because he failed to arrest anyone for months! He turned around and got sixty-one people in one day! He used to chase us in the Comrades too, but I ran away! Once he gave a citation to my mom!"

True love.

"He was born 1932 and Mom in 1932. We were living at his father's farm, but then we got moved—1987, I remember. I was thirteen and I just did my initiation school"—community rites of passage where girls may become young women. "We were paid 11,000 rand to move from the farm to the new place called Saselani. They were told that government made us move, and that they would be paid another installment, but it was never paid. Or maybe it's still coming. It was not enough because the new house we built was 25,000!"

On my own phone, I cannot find a historical conversion rate for the amount, but you know it wasn't a lot, of course.

Me: "You were forced to go?"—deducing that their farm was land they lived on that someone said suddenly no longer belonged to them. In whites' parlance, they were likely "squatting" and became a "burden" to some white plans for municipal expansion and development.

"It wasn't a matter of 'must,'" she explains. "If you wanted to stay, you could, but it was a problem to stay because," she starts laughing again, "we were afraid of

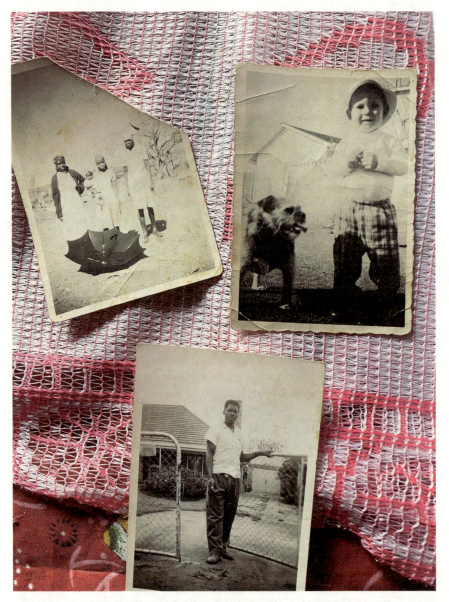
memories

electricity! We weren't used to living that way. We cooked with firewood from the Park, remember."

Electrification, an altogether new utility for many in the region, as part of whites' directed municipal expansion and development. Their farm became a "location," another word for a majority-black township outside of some white-centric place.

"He was soooo happy to retire from doing police," she exclaims of her father. By then, 1999, Gazankulu and the other homelands had been reabsorbed into South

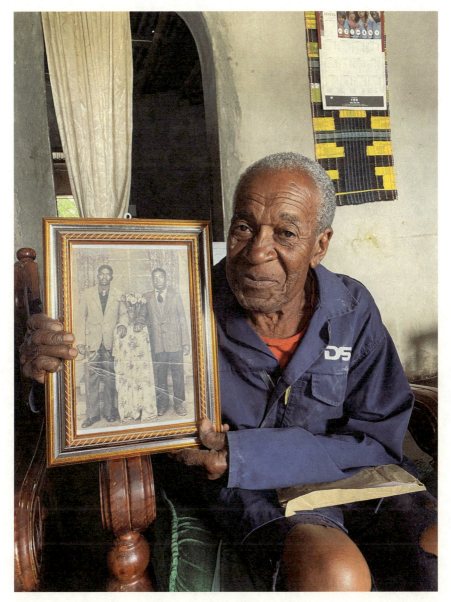

now and then

Africa, and their employees got a properly timed exit from the workforce, with pension, based on the new 1994 Public Service Act.

In Boston University's archives, I read some of Gazankulu's annual reports from the 1980s, from Goodness's and her grandparents' time, that social welfare and health care professionals in the homeland said elder care services were needed, but nothing was built.

"Would he have wanted to go to an old age home?" I ask.

"Never. It is difficult to move these older generations from their place. For my grandmothers, too, even when their husbands passed away. My gogo said to my mother, 'No, I can't go to live with you, my daughter-in-law! I didn't marry you! If someone wants to look after me, they must come here'"—meaning Goodness's grandmother decided to stay where she'd lived with her spouse, aging in place alone in their marital home, rather than move to live as a widow with her adult son and his wife—"But it was my mom who changed things. She was the one who went to an old age home!"

The one called Security. She told us about it before, but I'm still surprised by it.

"It's by the Park where I stay. Like I said, we'll go see it soon. My mom really told us she did not want to be a burden as she got older. At the time, my father wasn't around, and I was working, so Mom thought it was the best place for her to go."

"What was so burdensome?"

"She was getting dizzy working in the garden. We took her to Themba, and I think her soldiers were low. Her body was just not that good. She knew I worked here but heard me talk about Security. She surprised us, *nje!* She just told my sisters and me, 'Take me, please!' We laughed, like, 'Where did she get this idea?' Then Mom told us: 'If you don't take me there, I will call social welfare and say you're abusing me!'"

I laugh at Mom's cunning.

"I just told my sisters, 'Look, I know my mom, let her go. She won't like it and will want to come back.' So we went."

"How is Security different than Grace?"

"You'll see for yourself."

There may be time still on this tour. It's not even teatime yet, I think. The ladies sitting in here with us don't seem like they're waiting in under-caffeinated anticipation.

Like I asked Bethal, "Nowadays do you think it's more common for black families to have their parents in places like these?"

"I think so for some. Now they are educated"—Mama Zulu's kids or adult children of older adults, she means, and the social workers who saw it best for the abandoned ones like Miss Motsa and Mr. Xitangu. "They understand what a place like Grace means for old age. Way back then, they thought putting someone in here is like leaving them behind, but it's not that. And I think it's the same for the whites. No one's ignoring them. We're their confidants and Care Buddies!"

The real question though, "Would you want to be here or somewhere like it then?"

"Well," hesitatingly, "by then I will check my situation. Maybe where I am staying with my new husband, they will take care of me, but if not, I will go back to my family's home."

Sounds similar to her grandmothers' generation's preferences.

GOODNESS

And like her mother: "I just don't want to be a burden to anyone. I just want to sleep and rest. The righteous shall eat their fruits they say, and I use that when I think about who will help me and who I have helped."

I think I can hear the tea cart ambling across the tiles somewhere down the hall, and—eyeing these different women, black and white, sitting with us at the table, I ask her, "You help so many people here. Are they grateful?"

"They are, Casey, yes. Some try to be"—maybe trying to be less burdensome in their gratitude—"but some are not."

"What do you do if they say terrible things to you—racist things—or accuse you?"—of what, I don't say.

Earnestly, willing the voice of her father the Zionist pastor maybe, "I will look at them and quote the Bible verse that says, 'God created us all equal.' With the help of the Holy Spirit, *you* can see something is wrong with their situation. But with spiritual wisdom you can help to heal it and maybe move them to not do that next time. Other times they'll tell you things that happened in the past, things they once did to their family or others that were bad, or you hear them say racist things now. You see, for some it's just in their character."

"So they cannot change their behavior?"

"What I'm saying is that when some get older, they can't change that or control it. So, you just take good care. We can't overcome the past, so we must pray for better times. If you have three pieces of wood tied together, you can't just break one off with an axe. All of them will be chopped. So we must stand together, and united we conquer."

Let's bring the sermon to a close. None of the women we're watching drank from their bottles yet, but the tea is coming in hot.

"What is it that you would want us to know about all of this, your family, this place, what matters in the end?"

"Well, if you know you've wronged someone," she ends, "then make peace with them before you go. Forgive and ask for forgiveness. When the time comes, accept Jesus Christ and expose yourself to Him. You'll be forgiven for all those you have wronged without even knowing it. I think that's the best thing I've learned, and what I can tell you now."

I think I've learned something else, too.

That all racists are witches, but not the reverse, and both are possessed, captured perhaps, by evil, an ethically unjust or corrupt force that originates in human conditions[10]—much like white supremacy.

Witches—the ones who *do not* self-identify or self-affirm as such—are supposedly abnormal, immoral, or inhuman. You don't know you're a witch until it is something you're accused of or cursed upon you by people who are possessed by the aforementioned evil. Again, as in Salem, Massachusetts, or in Bushbuckridge, it is most often people with power, men or women, who accuse other women or the most vulnerable or marginalized in our communities as witches. When you come to realize you've been accused or cursed like this, cast as the scapegoat in a conspiracy or power play, there is little you can do to escape, even if you see the playing field clearly for what it is.

Racists themselves are also possessed, captured perhaps, by this evil. I think about those racist white women we call Karens (Karenijkies here maybe?) who also become a kind of witch.[11] When Karens are openly accused, "caught" for their racist remarks or assaultive actions, they become dislodged from their white privileged position. Dislodged from their obliviousness of the power they hold due to it. Shocked, perhaps, to now be accused by others of racism—itself the evil that's possessed them—of something they've said or done which to them felt just. Karens-as-witches cry, scream, denying others' accusation or curse upon them—they're broken. As clarity of their possession takes over, some grasp at color blindness— "it doesn't matter what color you are"—or claim someone's used the "race card" against them, excuses that ultimately fail to save face in the face of their situation.

They believe they'll die—not literally, but more like a temporary social death online. Burned at what they believe is the stake of anti-racist justice. Actually, they've been shown their possession by white supremacy, their unconscious collusion with the evil that has benefited them until it did not. Losing that benefit feels like mortal danger.

Still, racists aren't usually killed like witches are. Neither are sangomas—false or not—who might identify witches in the first place.

You may find yourself in danger when calling a white person a racist, however.

The cart with tea and condiments rolls into view at the end of the hall.

"Do you have any favorites?" I try to milk a last drop of gossip.

"The two I meant to sign up for. The two former police, Yvonne and Louw! Yvonne, though, when I first did my practicals she helped me with transport money to get to work. I bought her chocolates, and she did for me. She's a prayer warrior. We pray together."

Daughters of Christ, brandishing weaponry for battle—a cross for prayer, knives to cut bread rolls, a gun.

"She says she is like mother to me."

~

"Casey, I quit."

"Why, neh?"

"There were too many people. At night you run up and down and it becomes too hard to watch." On night shift at Grace, it's two caregivers like Goodness and the staff nurse, Janice, for the near-fifty souls. The care is subacute, but it's still a lot to do.

GOODNESS

I think again about Charlie—nights on a travel contract at a new mega-hospital in suburban Southern California. Gleaming windows, views of scrub brush, sunsets, private rooms for every in-patient versus the curtained partitions for two to four or more which is the usual. A Starbucks. A facade for a patient-as-client-as-hotel-guest suite.

The charge nurse would shunt the travel nurses first to a "special kind of Hell" in the mega-ER—the "off-load" line. It was that hospital's protocol to send off the ambulances quickly to return with more patients and leave the patients "off-loaded" and lined up in beds in a hall. In most hospitals, EMTs wait until the patient gets into an actual room with a bed. Some nights, he was the one nurse responsible for up to twenty off-loaded patients. In California, the unions fought for an ER nurse-to-patient ratio of one to three or four, depending on the role.

Nights were mad—running like crazy, doing some minimal thing, anything for each of the twenty souls lying queued there, waiting for a room. Some screaming, "No, help me" or trying to crawl out toward the dignity of a toilet rather than spoiling the gurney's thin sheet. Sometimes a room was never available. Patients would eventually be discharged from their hallway bed once a doctor eventually came around.

"It's poor care," Charlie told me.

"I'm an agent nurse now," Goodness says, "home-based care. I have just the one client."

She shows me a picture of a tannie on her phone, a suety white woman beaming in a recliner, a walker parked next to her.

"Basically, I change her, change her clothes, bathe, give the medication. All the same things at Grace, but I don't have twenty clients. The pay is good for just this one."

The little tannie lives on a "forest estate"—a lush term for a timber plantation—near one of the Park's gates. Mini-buses don't always run there so sometimes she stays with Pretty who lives nearby.

Sometimes she stays overnight with the little tannie,

Watching,

Waiting.

Jokers

"Ride the scale, mama."

It's the first of the month, or somewhere near it, which means blood pressure checks and weigh-ins. The tea cart's still making its rounds, and we want to get their numbers before they get their caffeine.

Most are going to take theirs with lots of white or brown sugars if the dietary recs permit it. Sometimes they do not. Friendly collusions mean bent rules.

"It just tastes better, neh," says Noeline.

Angel made a cute retching noise when I drank my coffee at this morning's diversity training without it. The nutritionist is on contract and hasn't been around for a few months, but we know the gist.

Precious and Gugu yoke me in to help them do a final pass with the clipboard in hand.

"He'll write fast for us."

We run room to room, cajoling residents to get on board the white metal plate that squeaks depressingly each time.

"And the accessories! Chic!"—a blue blood pressure monitor.

Anne's next. Through door crack, Precious's on her spy game.

"She's sleeping."

Gugu barges in. "Hey LaRoux, we are here to check on you!"

Anne turns over to her other hip. Precious massages the bony point under the blanket.

"You are not dreaming now, mama."

Precious laughs.

"It's Paul, you see, LaRoux. He's real! Tell us what he says so we go to the mountain with you to show us where to find the pot of money."

Are we dreaming of leprechauns? I guffaw. Precious howls. It's too ridiculous.

JOKERS 109

"Yeah, so?" Anne snaps, blinking more and rolling over.

Paul Kruger is the namesake for the nearby Park, itself a UNESCO Biosphere Reserve. Paul was the president of the Boer colonial South African Republic—its second version, 1881–1902, falling in war to the British. He established a mint in the wake of the region's major gold discoveries. Its coins became known to black locals as *imali lePawula* (Paul's money), or *imali letipoko* (ghosts' money). They believed that Paul's soldiers, fleeing the British, buried their gold coins—as well as humans as sacrifices—in caves and mountains to unearth them later. Others say the coins are the remains of what white businessmen paid the giant snake who dwells beneath the earth's crust to give them permission to mine for gold.[1] When the whites died or left the area, the wealth was free to take if you could find it. You only had to defeat the ghosts who hovered around the burial site.

Outside here, buried near Grace's front gate, are other ghosts who were once people—the buried relatives of Grandpa Malopa and his community, those who were left behind when their families were evicted by settlers who might also be long-distance relatives of Paul and his soldiers. They're still lying here, nearby the independent-living cottage units,

Listening, perhaps, to a resident's puttering footsteps upon her kitchen floor or patio.

I now wonder if the dementia and other afflictions of older people here are more than a biological condition.

Maybe they're being haunted.

Anne the sleeping beauty is still rising.

Gugu tugs on Precious's apron and we leave to measure Jane O. next door.

"Ooo-eechee!" the scale squeaks, depressed by the farmer's wife.

Back a few minutes later, Anne's doing the downward dog, her nightgowned derrière arched high in the air making a royal mockery of our pleas to take her basic health indicators.

"Come on, moonshine" says Precious.

"Christ, give me a few minutes."

"Come on, stand up!" Gugu touches her shoulder, and Anne gets up. "Ride the scale, mama!"

The light hand takes mine and mounts the scale. "Ooo-eechee!"

We wait for the little black analog number.

Lesego from the kitchen finally gets here with the tea cart and banana bread and her phone that plays Justin Bieber, then Nakhane Touré. The ladies talk like they haven't seen each other in years, laughing about someone's sorry-ass husband, ignoring us for a second. Their voices' reverb against the tiles is loud.

I think Anne's going to get more agitated—"Wow, they're noisy!"

She pats her knees like cakes and laughs, "It's like a pack of monkeys in here!"

I hope the ladies didn't hear that.

Precious puts the fashionably blue monitor around Anne's arm.

"I'm dead, right?" she says with each pump.

"You're a ghost!" laughs Gugu.

Charlie tells me when he draws a patient's blood and asks, "Do you need anything else?" one of the all-time favorite joking comebacks is "a million dollars!"

Or they call him a vampire.

I write down the blood pressure count on the clipboard fast as they made me promise.

Tea now! "*Cup iku'?*" (Where's your cup?) Gugu asks. They bend down to rummage through the bedside cabinet.

Lesego waves the teapot like a beer stein and hollers down, "Oh Annie, *bayangibita ngikhon' nje!*" (they're asking me if I'm OK!).

"*Bungalile tjwala, hieeeee!*" the others squeal. "Drinking is not good for me" are the siSwati lyrics and song title I find on the Smithsonian Folkways Recordings catalog, from 1958.[2]

Precious pulls out a mug with a reclining pink lion on it.

"LaRoux, *'tak'shay!'*" (I'm gonna beat you) laughs Gugu. "*Dit is Marina se beker*" (This is Marina's cup).

"What do you mean?" croaks Anne.

"She's stealing from us like a maid!"

Anne hides and hoards the dishes that come with meals or other things she finds around the home. Howie and Eunice do too. The aides get to be archaeologists and dig them up on their rounds.

She's not really going to beat her. It's just a joke to shape up, whether Anne can do it quite fully or not doesn't matter.

Lesego switches out the pink lion for one with yellow smiley face—*Forrest Gump*'s.

"Here's another, gogo."

~

Back down the hall in the sitting room is a big group—Mama Zulu, Miss Motsa, and Little Marie. Gugu, Bethal, and Goodness wheel in a few more residents—Barra (Beyoncé), Eunice, Howie, Nettie. Someone's blown up a balloon to bat around.

Another round of teacups and plastic plates for the banana bread.

"Drink, Mariejkie!" Precious slides down face-to-face with the scowler, throws her head back to show how.

"*Nee!*" (No!) laughs Mariejkie.

And "*Sawubona* (Hello), Janejkie" to Jane Zulu.

"I hate those 'kies,'" rumbles Gugu, the diminutives that get tacky-tacked onto everyone's name. Because if you're old you're also somehow an infantilized sweetie baby.

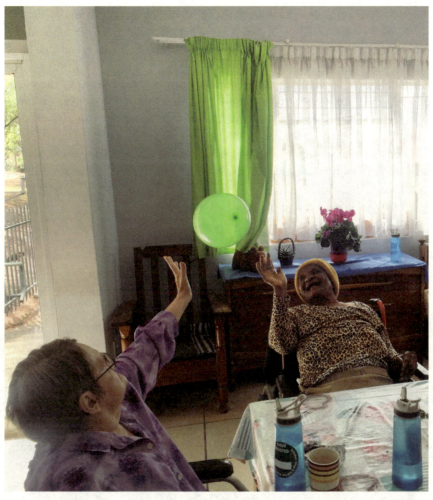

play

"*Ngiyafa mntanam'! Thela phela!*" (I'm dying, my child! Pour, pour!), laughs Mama Zulu.

"*Womile gogo*" (Grannie's thirsty), I say.

"Dry as bones!"

Nettie goes beady-eyed, asking me, "*Praat jy Afrikaans nie?*" (You don't speak Afrikaans?)

"Nettie, there's no Afrikaans in America. It's African," sighs Bethal.

Charlize Theron once said on a podcast the Afrikaans language was dying, as a joke.[3]

Howie knows siSwati really well. He used to evangelize all over the homelands. Precious jokes that he could be her new husband because he already knows how to *lobola*—that is, pay her family cash or cows so that she becomes his bride. He can use his monthly grants to pay. Some of the white residents are better at Fanagalo, that pidgin or creole language here that flourished in the mines among diverse black people who spoke their own diverse languages with each other and the English and Afrikaans of their white bosses. The white Sisters are earnest but don't get much beyond "sawubona" and "*ngithanda wena*" (I love you).

The multiple languages flying around is normal.[4] Crossed wires, the shock of what comes up, who says it and how, is all part of a joke. Jokes can be about figuring out what someone said, in whatever language, but you also need to "get it."

I don't want to tell you why things they're saying are funny. If you're not from here, you probably won't get it. You won't hear another layer of meaning in the exchange,

Or maybe because your hearing aid battery is dying.

"Nettie, your husband is coming today," snickers Gugu.

The beady-eyed woman jumps in her seat, "Oh! Really?"

"Oh yes, he's coming to take you to town. I bet you go shopping!"

"Oh! Oh!" she huffs, bouncing under her bib. She looks like she's revving to lift off. Va-va-va-voom!

"Nettie's my favorite performer. She's my Shakira," says Precious.

"Waka waka, eh eh!"

Performers are those stars of Grace who do the fabulous, the strange, the surprising and unexpected. You don't even need to buy a ticket—they pay you to work here and you get to see it. When they take the stage, so to say, their outbursts leave the staff multiply confused, angered, or genuinely bowled over. An angering performance might be when a resident throws her feces out of her window, as Linda told me had happened last week. A wild one might be this dance-bounce, the oontz-oontz-oontz you do if you know your husband's coming.

The caregivers are howling.

Eunice mutters, pushing the crust of the banana bread around the plate, "Her husband has been dead a long time." Barra's eyes dart to Eunice, then to me, asking, "What's going on?" I think she asks that because it is now loud with the caregivers laughing and Nettie bouncing, "Oh! Oh!"

"She knows her husband's coming!" laughs Precious.

Lesego pours two sugars, three sugars, four sugars, five sugars—now it's really going to get wild.

Nettie rewinds for another go, asking me the same but now as her brother, "Praat jy Afrikaans nie, *boetie*?"

"Nettie! *Hy is nie Afrikaner nie!*" (He's not an Afrikaner!).

"It's a European language too," I offer.

"Jan van Riebeeck came from someplace like that in the 1900s," says Gugu—the European corporate pioneer who first settled a commercial port for the Dutch East India Company in the seventeenth century as a colonial outpost in what is today Cape Town. Gugu's off by about three centuries, but who's counting. "He gave us the mirror," she continues, "we got the mirror and they took the cattle!"

JOKERS 113

That was a raw deal, something of no real value—a tool for vanity versus the materially and economically sustainable beasts you use for lobola, milk, and the plow.

"That was our wealth," instructs Bethal.

It reminds me of a vision well known by Swati people. King Sobhuza I, or Somhlolo (his second name can mean "miracle") had a deathbed vision that white-skinned people with hair like cow's tails appeared from the dreamy mists to offer a disc or a scroll.

Somhlolo chose the scroll—symbolizing written law, the Bible, an interpretive rubric for authoritarian governance, other text messes, it depends on who you ask— rather than the disc—which was money, maybe the prototype of a gold Kruger coin.

"What about the land?" I ask.

That's been a black South African Twitter/X favorite. If you're white and make a funny, you can keep the piece of land you got unfairly, they say. They won't take it back.

"First the cattle, then the land," Gugu clarifies, "Our gogos were stupid, neh, they took the mirror, but we already had the river. Just look down in water to see yourself!"

The staff laugh some more. Both sides, white and black, be damned, honestly.

"It was our wealth," Bethal says again.

"Our inheritance!" says Goodness.

"What can you say, neh," says Gugu. Then looking over and pointing at Nettie, "I bet it was *you!*"

Her finger's rigid like an arrow aimed at the white woman wearing too little foundation to cover her liver spots, clip-on pearl earrings, and a bib tucked into the neck of her blouse.

Here's something like the punchline:

Rereading the essay "The Case for Reparations" by Ta-Nehisi Coates, I came across a line where he writes that "the popular mocking of reparations as a hare-brained scheme authored by wild-eyed lefties and intellectually unserious black nationalists is fear masquerading as laughter."[5]

In the American context, Coates means that when typically-conservative whites laugh at blacks who claim economic reparations for slavery and its aftermath, it's a fearful reflex. They believe that reparations could actually happen—another white anxiety.

At Grace, as on social media and in public life in South Africa, it is blacks like Gugu and Precious who laugh at whites who are in the minority. A series of humorous jabs that could conjure a sense of dignity or equality in the meantime, while another series of more substantive legal actions aim to restore something more material:

Land—like Grandpa Malopa and the community are fighting for, less jokingly so. Land on which Nettie, or rather her adult children and grandchildren and other whites in postcolonial countries, remain steadfast even if they feel increasingly uncertain about their bids to belong.[6] Still, none of the staff here told me they'd eventually try to take back the land or anything else from Nettie, her children, or whites in general. Nor try to nationalize the country's natural resources or systems like health care to uplift the black majority like the EFF desires.

Maybe they just haven't told me because I'm also white.

Maybe you think these jokes aren't funny at all. That they are unfair or abusive, or they don't even sound like jokes. (I guess we should have hired Trevor Noah and his writers.)

The critics Lauren Berlant and Sian Ngai wrote that a new, "youthful" generation has "new normative constraints" which police aspects of comedy they deem unconscionable in favor of intersectional sensitivity and historical redress.[7] This youthful generation is the antithesis to jokers who are glossed as outdated, conservative, or of another era, the ones who tend to say that "people just can't take a joke anymore." Their jokes also tend to be heard as racist, sexist, and ableist. We mostly let ageist ones slide for some reason.

Maybe for the so-called Rainbow Nation, these jokes and off-color humor both reveal and suture cracks or divisions among the country's citizens in the aftermath of apartheid's racial violence. Some of the joking you heard today might sound racist, sexist, ableist, and ageist, yes. And none of these angles would work without the others. Altogether, this kind of joking rearticulates usually problematic discourses, but in doing so, it also makes otherwise taboo topics speakable, argues literary scholar Grace Musila.[8] Topics like racism, sexism, and the like that we must be conscious of and talk about.

These are topics that some politicians try to curtail or altogether eliminate in American public schools, in places like Florida or where I work in New Hampshire.

Maybe off-color humor here is itself a shade of Black.[9]

In Grace, joking brings people together who have otherwise been historically primed to despise each other across the generations. Joking is a language of sorts that carves out an alternative place and time to talk to each other—an Elsewhere, perhaps. But I guess that's what we've known for a long time about a joke. It's cathartic (lets off steam) among oddly positioned groups of people who might otherwise be equals at certain moments in the right place and time: a place like God's waiting room.

And again, maybe by joking with old racists now—by meeting them halfway in some twisted humor before they pass on and become ancestors or ghosts—is one way to prevent them from haunting us later.

I don't think the target of Gugu's finger-arrow will be easy to hit. It's not Nettie herself, and it's not black-and-white or colorfully cut like the prism of a dart board.

JOKERS

It's a gray zone, rather, a point of oblivion,
A plate of crumby banana bread.
Confusion.

"What is going on?" asks Nettie.

"She says you know Jan van Riebeeck," I say. "Do you really think she is *that* old, Gugu?"

We laugh.

Yvonne

"I lived the war. I mean I *lived it*. The bullet lying in my lap was when I realized God saved my life for a purpose."

"I told you, she's full of gold."

Paul Kruger's gold, maybe? Angel's told us this woman, Yvonne, is good for plenty of stories and apparently told her that we'd come to talk to her on the tour. Angel's just brought us from the A wing comedy hour to meet her specifically.

White-blond Yvonne wears mother-of-pearl cat-eye frames and sits in one of the elevated chairs behind her "little carriage" (*karretjie*). On her walker's tray lies a mobile phone, an adult coloring book—the ones with dastardly complex stained glass window-like images that are supposed to help you relax into mindfulness or mindlessness—a box of crayons, a room key.

No bullet,

Yet.

She's getting situated by waving away two black teenage girls in plaid skirts. Once in a while, the nearby posh boarding school sends students like them down to do meet-and-greets. Today, they're doing a survey about the residents' quality of life and transportation access.

She's not amused.

"These questions are all in Afrikaans. I'm British. And don't you see there aren't any cars out in the parking lot?"—none of the residents drive.

"We have the form in English too," one girl says, undeterred.

"Quit bothering me! Don't you see I'm already busy talking to this one."

Me.

"He's American. So we're talking in English."

That excites the girls more than their survey. To me: "What's it like there?" "How's New York?" "My mom's been to DC"—other quick-fires—"Let me take a picture of you both." "Yes, I know how to use an iPhone." "No, use portrait mode."

YVONNE

Louw scares them off after the shot. "Do you think something's wrong with speaking Afrikaans?" he barks.

No, we say. They move on.

He sneezes and moves on, bewildered by what's come out of his nose.

The TV's playing National Geographic. The room's just harassed him to change the channel from the weekly rugby recap. An anxious soundtrack with a rolling high-hat shimmer and explosions that would fit an action-thriller's car chase scene overlays a show about cheetahs.

A single mother, arching its haunches, ready to fire off the chase—prey. The kill is quick.

Angel's gone again.

The ladies watching in the room with us sigh—survival of the fittest.

"So," I ask her, "how?"—did she live the war, know the bullet meant something more? People with near-death experiences or those who are near others' deaths find they're changed somehow by the mortal encounter.

"Rhodesia," she begins.

The former British colony, then a white-settler nation-state, both named for the capitalist and imperialist Cecil Rhodes. (He who must fall in image, statue, and legacy, the new generation argues.) The war there, from 1964 to 1979 by most historical accounts, where black peoples who found themselves living within the new borders of this Southern African country. With help from the Chinese, Soviets, and other black African countries, they fought for liberation from white-minority rule to become the new country of Zimbabwe.

"Let me tell you," she continues. "My husband and I moved up near the mines—Chimanimani—which border Mozambique. It was all forest estates."

Around here it is blue gumtree or conifer plantations besides citrus and macadamia.

"We had many dogs and cats, but there were no animals up there like we saw on safari, never elephants or lions or anything like that. Anyway, Dennis worked on the diesel equipment for the estates. The war started while we were up there. It was a small community. And we lost a lot of friends because of what was happening."

"Which was . . ." I try to lead.

"They were coming over the mountain."

"'They' being . . ."

"The terrorists,"

In her mind, Robert Mugabe, politicians like Joshua Nkomo, others who first negotiated with the white settlers for graduated political inclusion and then turned against it, who decided to accelerate their liberation and were then detained. This all partially led to the war. Though dead now, Mugabe still lives rent-free in the heads of most white Rhodesians and in the main historical narrative about their former country.

"One Christmas we went to go see my sister in Bulawayo," she continues. "It happened midday. It was an ordinary sunny day. We were about sixteen kilometers outside of Chimanimani. My husband was driving, and my son was sitting behind him. He was thirteen years old. And as we came around the border, all hell let loose."

On my neck, the show's soundtrack crescendos to the sound of searing metal.

"They always go for the driver first before they ambush you. Take out the driver and then kill the others. When they started firing, my husband started zig-zagging because he knew what to do. My son and I fell to the floor, to where you put your feet under the console."

My mouth's agape and likely keeps her going.

"He managed to drive us out of the ambush. I could hear bullets hitting the road. When we got away, I saw that bullets had come through the window and the sides of the car. When I got up, I saw the shrapnel hanging from my leg. I saw I was bleeding from somewhere else. My son looked into my eyes, and said, 'Mom . . .'

There, and there."

She gestures to her face with her pointer and middle fingers.

Under her powdery foundation, you can see a faint scar along her forehead, another along her cheekbone. Each an almost perfect graze, the kind of well-placed scar leading actors get from a Hollywood makeup team, rather than a more hideously real, imperfect disfigurement that war typically reckons upon the body.

On her other hand, on the ring and pinky fingers, there's nothing left above her metacarpals.

"When I looked down, on my lap was a bullet."

The revelation.

"We kept driving, further down the road to the army camp. They gave me tea to calm me. And some went back to see if they could find the ones who ambushed us. Who knows what they found? We should have gone to the hospital, but it was closed for two more days because of Christmas"—for Boxing Day, I guess, or maybe just short-staffed like hospitals are today. "We went on to my sister's with shrapnel hanging out of my face. We couldn't just pull it out."

Some present.

"There was nothing else to do."

Just wait.

"It was a quiet Christmas after that. On the Monday we made it to the hospital, finally. They did X-rays, took out what they could. They showed me the pieces that remained, just three tiny, minute pieces, and a few in my back. They eventually came out of me, just fell out when I slept."

Self-healing by some gentle power.

"They told me that I was really lucky to be alive."

"I can't imagine. I would've been terrified."

She scoffs, "I wasn't. I was used to gunfire because of the way I lived. I carried a weapon on me always."

I wonder how they compared to Goodness's firearms.

And like Goodness, "I never actually fired it," she says, "'twas a small pistol, but I learned to. We had to. We were alone up there. My son was at boarding school in Umtali"—Mutare. "My nearest neighbor was five kilometers away."

The quietude of the woods, waiting for someone who might never come.

"And my husband was in the army, in for a month and back out for two weeks holiday R&R and back. He came and went. So, I carried a weapon. The clearance came from the police for things related to what I did for the army and for the DC. They had a special thing connected to the police called an "Agric Alert." I manned that at the DC office and police station too. They gave me permission to use an automatic shotgun, but like I said, I never fired it."

I've seen DC—shorthand acronym for "District Commissioner"—in colonial-era papers of archives I've been to. Alerts were delivered and monitored as part of radio work for the regional command center of the Rhodesian Security Forces' Combined Operations program, the coordinated efforts of the white-settler nation's army, air force, and police forces that fought the "terrorists."

"So, that's why I carried the weapon," she explains. "We had to return to the forest estates and stayed there a while, but things got more dangerous. Then we moved to Melsetter. It was a small village, but it's where the DC was. There was a hotel and one of those old shops that sold everything, from nails to you name it. It was lonely there too, the nearest proper food shop was still a hundred kilometers away, where my son stayed for school."

"So you were with Ian Smith's people?"—the then president of Rhodesia.

"Yes. I was in the reserve, actually, and," more quietly, "part of the secret staff. My proper job was in that little village office, but on weekends I'd go to Chapinga, about forty kilometers from there, and worked the army radio."

"But why fight? Was it for your 'home' of Rhodesia? So they"—the terrorists—"wouldn't take it?"

The historian Luise White asked the same question of other white Rhodesian soldiers like Yvonne's husband. She argues things were different for them in their war against black people compared to the "great wars"—World Wars I and II—that dominate what we think we know about world history. The men of those great wars went to battle with "war-in-the-head," to use terms of World War II veteran and literature professor Samuel Hynes. That meant the men went off to fight in the great wars with big ideas that it would be fantastically heroic in a mission accomplished by total victorious control of the enemy.[1]

I think of a World War I saga I watched on Netflix with Charlie. The maybe-fictional German General Friedrichs sends his regiment back to the trenches fifteen minutes before the November 11, 1918, 11:00 A.M. armistice because of his undying pride. Wine-drunk, he slurs that his father was a soldier in the Otto von

Bismarck years.[2] Bismarck's years and the military of his generation carved up Africa cartographically at the Berlin Conference of 1884–1885, and then later went on massacre black African peoples like the Herero in what is today Namibia, the first genocide of the twentieth century.[3] In the film, Friedrichs moans that he'll never see victories for the *Vaterland* as he should.

German critics said the film was the worst-ever adaptation of Erich Maria Remarque's famous novel by the same name in its English translation, *All Quiet on the Western Front.* In the United States, it received nine Oscar nominations.[4]

People love war,

Or maybe men do.

In contrast, Luise White says the white Rhodesian soldiers she met didn't have the same imagined daddy issues as great war soldiers. War was not an expected victory bestowed to them from their forefathers. In Rhodesia, rather, they fought a "war-in-place," shaped by racist ideas of the African "bush" they'd settled in. Many knew they'd never be able to govern it, nor be victorious, but still envisioned it could be some non-black Elsewhere for themselves. In the memoirs of these men, White learned, many wrote about how this feeling grew inside of them by growing up and playing with black peers in their childhood.

Maybe the love of place, a settled life in the "bush" after a lifetime of moving, is what rooted Yvonne's fight.

Again, she scoffs, "No, I was bored! I needed something to do! The husbands were away, so you got to see all the wives and everyone else you went down to work on the weekends. Remember, it was lonely up there."

Other white women like her felt the same.[5]

"Mugabe promised the terrorists that they would each get a white woman," she says she heard somewhere, "so you better know that we went to fight! We stayed in Melsetter until the end of the war and then came to South Africa. I did tell you that we lost a lot of people. And that was over forty years ago. I'm now eighty."

What would *you* say to her so far, right now?

(Go away, colonizer.)

Face-to-face, scars and all, with some sincerity actually, I find myself saying, rather, "You're so brave."

"I fear nothing because I have God inside in me. But He wasn't always there. The war is where I learned to find the Lord. To look for the good things in people, to do what I could for them. He came into me then, but it took time to learn and accept things as they are."

The bullet,

A revelation.

"I wasn't a nice person, Casey. Some would tell you I was terrible, like that first husband of mine. But that Christmas day, I knew God had blessed me."

~

YVONNE 121

"You lived the war; the way you lived your life was changed by it."

"I was born from it! Or reborn. It makes sense to me as God's plan. I am a war baby, after all."

"You said British, yes?"

"By birth, yes, in Bristol—1939, just after the war started"—World War II— "Things were bad then in England and Australia. With everything going on, my father was recruited for a job here. He was a retort setter, used to lay bricks to build factories' steam towers. He is someone who can't stay in one place for very long. He's what they call a wandering stone."

Part of a generation of white Europeans—demobilized soldiers, tradesmen, their families—who were enticed to Southern Africa for economic prosperity and then partially enveloped in white Southern Africans' nationalist projects to modernize their minority-ruled, settler-colonial territories.[6]

And the fragments that break away from the stone and roll along with it?

"My mother and sister and I followed him a year later—1947. My sister is five years younger than me, seventy-five now. The last year before we came here, we stayed with my grandparents. Very strict people. My grandmother was one of thirteen children and kept things in order. My grandfather was very, very strict with us. I was happy we left. First to Grahamstown, then Port Elizabeth, and then Cape Town. I went to many schools in Cape Town. I mostly grew up there."

"Were things better in South Africa than Bristol?"

"I don't know, really"—and how could she? "I was really young then, so you don't really take notice. I had a good life there. But here, my mother was the main trouble for us.

"How so?

"My mother got cancer while we were in Cape Town, and she was in the hospital for eighteen months. My father had to put us in a home while he went to work to bring in money."

So it's not her first time she's come to a place like Grace, someplace where others take care of you—an institution.

"It was actually three different homes, I remember now. For children. Both my sister and I. People looked after us there, but we had to pay rent. It wasn't free. After that, for school, he used to give me bus money to take the train from Rondebosch to Observatory to school. By age sixteen, I was at my last school there, in Obs."

And your mother?

Flatly: "She recovered, but she was never the same. That was when they first discovered cancer, and they didn't know what they know today about it or how to cure it."

They still do not, prayerfully or medically, but it is better—"Were you close to her?"

"Yes. Well . . . my father died first and then my mother." Again hesitatingly, "They were a loving couple. I mean everybody has their fights and ups and downs, you know. Um . . . we got along together."

Pausing, we listen to the National Geographic narrator explain that female and male cheetahs only mix to mate.

"Was your father just as strict?" like his own father, I wonder.

"He was a firm person. We were brought up knowing right is right and wrong is wrong. There is no in-between. I didn't do a little white lie. But my parents were good to us. We were looked after. We knew they had the money to support us, to put us in the homes and school. The last of my girl years were in Bechuanaland. Do you know what Bechuanaland is today?"

I do.

"Botswana, but then it was a British protectorate. There were British police and services, but not much else I recall."

Besides Tswana people and other peoples who've been there for millennia.

"Only dirt roads. It was like that film *Out of Africa!*"—Meryl Streep was a headliner on that one. "My father was recruited by their government to build quarantine camps for foot-and-mouth disease. My family all moved while I was completing the last year of school in Obs. They left. And I followed."

The wandering stone.

"I took the train all the way, alone! When I arrived, I found they had a large home, six or eight buildings. My father wanted me to stay close by to Setsikamma, where we were. So I finished my schooling at the capital then, Mafikeng."

At a convent, run by the Sisters of Mercy. I imagine colonial nuns to have also been a strict bunch.

"There was nothing merciful about them," she laughs, "I almost became one! They were strict and because I was around those rules and things, you get used to it. I gave it some thought, but it was not for me in the end. I would go to worship at the Methodists and other places instead. It was God's plan that I kept going."

Life cannot be all toil for the hereafter.

"I do fondly remember my school holidays, the time away from the sisters. They were so lovely. I sat on the back of a five-ton truck and went from one end of Falmouth right to the top of the Makurekure pans, all the way up to where all the game is. I love a safari."

National Geographic's now playing a washing powdered soap commercial. I think I once read that wild animals are more likely to be confused or repelled by us, rather than attack us as prey, because of the artificial scents of such products that hang on us from bathing.

"I had a really good life that way. After that was when I went up to Rhodesia, to Bulawayo with my sister. I've seen a lot of things."

"And you met your husband there?

"Yes, the first one, Dennis, the one I met in Bulawayo. We stayed there for a long time, seven years, where I worked for Standard Bank as a secretary in the insurance division. I even got certificates for learning how well to do the work there. That was before moving up to Salisbury, which is now Harare, and then to Chimanimani. After the war, we left."

They had to.

"We had to. I mean, in Zimbabwe, I mean Rhodesia, we ended up poor. We could hardly take out any money, and we lost a lot on the way out. I gave away a lot of my furniture. They were after those of us who were in the police and in the army. We came to South Africa then, to stay near the coal mines outside of Rustenberg. I worked in the office and my husband was a mechanic foreman, so we did really well. Life carried on, but after some time we got divorced."

"And your son?"

"That child of my own," the one on the floor of the car, shielded from the bullet and shrapnel, "he left for England. I don't see him often now," she says coolly.

Nameless.

"I was blessed by God with another son, the one I got later who helped to put me here"—in Grace—"he's not my biological son. He's my stepson. I brought him up from the age of eight. He's the one that looks out after me today. Alexandros."

Whose son is he?

"After Dennis, I met my second husband whose name I kept—Constantinides— he's not alive today. He was a Cypriot Greek, not South African. We met in Rustenberg, married for thirty years. Mr. Constantinides always wanted a café. I didn't!" she laughs.

"One of my favorite spots to relax," I say.

"It was in Naboomspruit. He bought it from his friend, and we ran it for five years. But they built the new highway to far from the town, and it moved all the traffic away from there, so it wasn't making for good business."

Like Silverdays, the sister home to Grace, killed by development, or isolation.

"We shut it and moved near here."

"Is he still with us?"

"No," apathetically, "we got divorced. He went back to Cyprus. He remarried and then got very ill. He died about five or six years ago."

"And Alex?" I shorten her stepson's name.

"He was older by then and didn't go with his father. He has his own business now, vending for the hotels. They had a contract for the All Blacks (the rugby team) when they came to play here last year! Alex has looked after me and pays for me here. He's not a child of God in the strong sense, but I know the Lord knows him still, if you know what I mean. He's really a good son. He's got two children—he's got a boy who's in his varsity in Pretoria and a daughter whose finishing up this year at Uplands"—the posh school those two girl surveyors came from.

Not to discomfort her, but two marriages, three countries, I ask, "How did you do it? You had to have been strong to go through those changes."

She seems a bit discomforted.

"Well, I know I have strength in me—God, my heart. I don't believe in letting myself get down by other people's issues. I made a life for myself. So, when Alex's father married another wife, God told me, 'This is what it is.' I had to forgive him."

The same for Precious, Goodness, other women and widows here who've been betrayed.

"And what advice would I give to people in a new relationship?" she responds to the question, "Never give up! You have to put in the work getting to know your partner. None of us are perfect, and some partners are more difficult than others, of course. I get stronger as I get older. I go by the grace of God."

To change the tone, let's ask where else she's gone—traveling, holidays, the like.

"Alex's father and I went to Greece and Sweden because he had a brother there. And Cyprus of course. It is a wonderful place. They have those tavernas and you can sit out and eat for hours."

The nostalgia for their little café. Maybe Angel could draw some inspiration for it too for her double-decker-bus coffee shop.

"It's not like here, where you have one meal and go. You can sit for hours because the weather is so lovely, enjoying that brandy liqueur. They loved spending the whole evening like that. You'll have to go. It was also where the South African doctor who did the first heart transplant died. Did you know that?"

Wikipedia tells me that Dr. Christian Barnard passed away from asthma there in 2001 while on vacation at age seventy-eight.

"After a while, though, you get tired of traveling around. When you get to my age you just want peace and quiet. I wouldn't like to travel today with the hassles of what's going on."

"And what kinds of hassles are those?"

"Just listen to the news, man. You can get on a plane today and don't know if it's going to get hijacked. You get in a taxi, and you don't know if you're going to get home safe. You might end up dead on the other end! What's going on in the world today is the end times. The beginning of the end. Those people who are not saved are going to have a big problem because if they don't know Jesus, they are going to Hell; they aren't going anywhere else. There's no halfway up."

"Even during the war, do you think it was safer back than it is now?"

"Yes, because during the war years, it took longer for us to know anything. Whether this place had been bombed or that place had been bombed. You heard on the telephone and the radio. It's not like what it is today, where within minutes the world knows because of your remotes and all: modern technology."

We still have to change the channel on the sitting-room TV in here by hand. There's more safety in ignorance. Less stress, I guess. "It's scary," I say, referring more to my own ignorance of how it all works.

"We would always say, as old people, that we come from the old times, not the new times. I don't have a modern cellphone as you can see," patting the little plastic brick on her walker. "I don't want all the rubbish they put on it."

Same, Yvonne. I hate downloading business's apps. I mean, like for Panera Bread or Mochachos—do we really need an app?

"They are always trying to get your money, stealing this and stealing that. I don't need that in my life."

"Is there anything you would do differently now that you look back on your life?"

She's quick to answer: "No. I don't look back on things, I don't regret anything. What's happened, happened. There is nothing for you living in the past because whatever you had can be gone in a moment."

YVONNE 125

Your home and material things, your loved ones,

You.

Louw is staring blankly ahead. Gugu and Linda are paired with Little Anne and Anne LaRoux in Care Buddy chat.

"And what of Grace? Do you like it?"

"I find it just fine, but you've found people moaning all over the place, I'm sure."

That's not what I've found or heard per se—"In pain, you mean?"—The first public hospital in the United States, Mass General in Boston, founded in the preanesthesia era, staged its operating room on the top floor, higher to Heaven, so to air the patients' cries away from the passersby on the street.

"You know, of life on earth. This is Mother Earth. And it will never be 100 percent A-OK. You will find fault with everything if you look for it hard enough. The only one place that there's no problem is up there"—her three full fingers point to the ceiling—"So until you get up there, just make the most of what you've got here. Half the people in this place don't realize how well-off they are. You should see the waiting list to get in. Someone has to die in order for it to happen."

She knows how Angel works.

"I was on the list myself. When Mr. Constantinides and I moved to White River, my stepsister-in-law also moved and bought a house. He took everything from me when I he left—car, the furniture, a place to live—and she helped me. I was blessed but couldn't stay there for long. She came to Grace to make inquiries. And I heard same thing."

Like I said before. It doesn't matter who you are. You have to wait.

And what did Angel say?

"'Oh, bring her,' she told her, 'we will interview her and everything, but there's a long waiting list.' I just said, 'OK, let's go and see.' I knew it could take six months or a year, depending on what happens. So I came for the interview. I was sitting right over there"—the waiting room—"and she came and talked to me one-on-one, without my stepsister-in-law. After that, right then and there, she said,

'Alright, you can move in tomorrow!'

'But I thought I'm on the waiting list?' I asked her.

'No worries, sweetie,'"—I guess one of Angel's favorite endearment terms—"'it's sorted.'"

"I really moved in two weeks later because I had to clear out the flat and everything by my stepsister-in-law. So I don't complain. The rest here moan about the food, their rooms, the cold, and moan about the taste of the water. We all go through the same thing, but no moaning is going to fix it. I know that elderly people like to. I am one myself! But when the Sisters greet me, they say, 'You're the only person who doesn't moan in this place,' and I say, 'I know.'"

And to me, before she takes a quick break to the bathroom, "Go to my room, you'll find *it* next in my side table."

C wing. No roommate. Lucky for her, but it's probably what she and the family pay for.

On the wall, framed pictures of white domes above the sapphiric Mediterranean, a cross of inlaid stained glass.

I open the bedside drawer to look in—a glass ashtray,

A bullet.

~

Back in the sitting room, now lying in her palm after I lay it there,

"I had it encased in silver."

(Yesterday is history, tomorrow is a mystery, but today: a present.)

"I am blessed," she says again. "God is good, and no place is always A-OK. So if I hear someone moaning, I say to them, 'You don't like it here? Pack your bags. There's the door. People are waiting to get in.'"

I hate the "get out and go if you don't like it here" attitude, because if we don't complain, rage, negotiate, or mobilize for change, nothing ever will. Still, she makes me laugh imagining she'd help kick anyone to the curb.

(She and the other white Rhodesians did it to others, of course, and they were shown the door.)

"Did you have people in your life there, like these ladies, like Goodness or Linda?"

"There were people who came and cleaned for us in the estates. We had big fences, but I was not nervous that our cleaners were terrorists. Is that who you mean?"

Maybe.

Bethal and Precious have joined Linda and Gugu with their Anne Care Buddies.

"And Goodness is your Buddy?" She's somewhere else on duty still.

"She is my favorite caregiver. She's been here for some time now. She prays with me, treats me well. She told me that I'm her second mother."

I draw out more from her eyes at that corroborating statement, their mutual truth.

"Yes, I believe she would say it. On Mother's Day, she brought me chocolates, even. She is good to me."

Like a daughter, a sister to Alex—he probably would not call her one—another child to replace the nameless son.

"Blacks are counted here, more than the coloured," she adds, "and I'll keep my voice lower here on this"—she both says and does with a hand to her mouth—"but I believe that most whites in here have a thing against the blacks. If I see them acting crazy or angry to one of the nurses, I let them know. I pull them aside to another room and speak softly to them and say, 'What if you were born black? How would you like to be treated?' No one likes to get picked on in front of people, and color doesn't matter. God loves us all, and I do too: black, yellow, or purple."

Again, let's hope there aren't any purple ones here. Everyone's got some kind of health care degree or certificate and helps to keep the blood flowing.

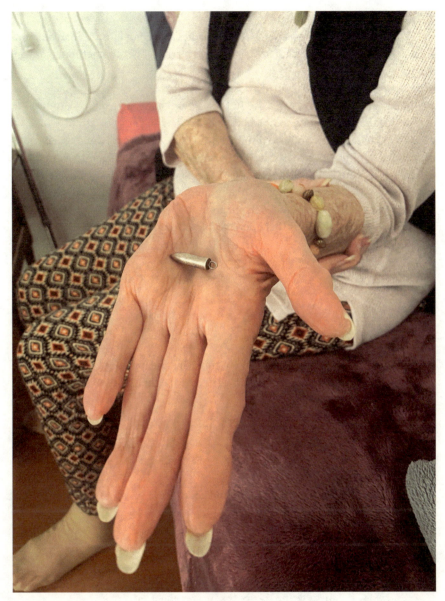

bullet

"Well, that perspective is important," I add, "because we've had the same issues in America"—old racists berating nursing staff of color.

"Look at the Ku Klux Klan by you in America, I mean, mama mia! I see that all on TV, and it doesn't make sense to me. How can you treat people like that? I'll tell you that everything we do, God sees. I've made mistakes in my life, and I go on knowing this. You must always treat others like you want to be treated. So that's my story."

128 GOD'S WAITING ROOM

"No moaning, no groaning."

"Like I said, you should see some of these ladies that complain, but maybe some of them really need to. Look at Barra, her hair is terrible! That's something to moan about!"

Shame, as they say.

"Like I said, Casey, you can't live in the past or change it. You have to live for today. I see that with a lot of old people in here who are angry or afraid. We are a spirit living in a human body, so if the body gives up tomorrow, there's no need to worry. If you think on the past, the pain, you won't go on. You have to want it, the will to live. And to have purpose. If I had one piece of advice for someone facing the end, I'd say, 'Never give up!'"—like in a new relationship—"Find the will to live, and want to live each day. With purpose. And at this point, I know what this is. If I do have a problem, it is that I don't fear anything. Because when I die, I know where I will be going."

Just be ready.

~

National Geographic is over. Noeline's come in and put on a DVD—*Andrea Boccelli Live in Central Park*. The camera pans over the thousands of souls obscured in New York City's twilight,

The sitting room hushes itself for an aria,

"Nessun Dorma":

"None shall sleep, even you,
Oh princess, in your cold room.
Watch the stars that tremble with love and hope,
But my secret is hidden within me,
My name no one shall know,
No . . . no . . .
On your mouth, I will tell it,
When the light shines.
And my kiss will dissolve the silence that makes you mine.
Vanish, oh night.
Set, stars!" twice, Andrea sings,
"At dawn, I will win."

Next to us, Louw's eyes begin to water. Passing the bullet from her hand to mine, Yvonne whispers,

"They will play this song at my funeral."

God

"I thought the next time I'd see you would be in Heaven!"

A bold statement from another sexy man—Father Matt, here for the weekly workshop service, a full house as usual—singling out Jane O. It's the first time she's been out of her room this week, oxygen tank in tow.

"I'm joking, but we know it was serious for you, Jane," he says. "You've been in a very dangerous state for a while, so I want to be truthful."

Everyone agrees, including Jane.

Grace is supposed to be nondenominational, taking in the white, black, yellow, and purple of every faith. But if you look in any direction, all you see are crosses on the walls, rustic style "God is *liefdie*" (love) signs like the ones that say "Live-Laugh-Love," Bibles aplenty in the library, and other stuff that has the holy aura of a plug-in nightlight.

Barra is at the piano—it's usually Miss Frikkie, Precious tells me. Someone's already passed out the bilingual hymnals.

"Some others, too, I'm so happy to see again—Trish, Johnny," some others like Jane O. who aren't so well. Each nods or waves a little. "Some of the services I did for you over the holidays were sparsely attended. I wonder if those of you who went to the Park instead of coming to worship did not see any animals!"

There's a wave of chuckles at the thought of their trips to Kruger being God-damned to miss seeing something astonishing like ten baby elephants. Anyway, none of the people he mentioned went on our safari. They probably stayed in their rooms—too frail to go out.

"Let's move to the sermon. I'm reading from Ephesians. You can remember the order of books in this part of the Bible by saying 'Gentiles Eat Pork Chops'—Galatians, Ephesians, Philippians, Corinthians. I know you will understand what I'll preach about today. You can hear"—understand—"God's Word because you're already made in the image of His son. It's natural like that."

Again, *Imago dei* theology, and I wonder how inclusive they knew they could be, if they knew that Bethal or Andrew also saw themselves in this way.

"Life is not a bed of roses, and we are blessed to live our lives because of Him. Still, we still live with problems. Maybe not like you see on the news with heroin or abortion. We know there are problems out there, but I don't know who is getting abortions in here! Or doing heroin, but I know nurses hold onto some good drugs back there!"

More laughter.

"I'm talking about things I know you all face. Like bitterness. Anger. Gossip. Will you raise your hand if you know what I'm talking about?"

No laughter, and no hands this time.

"I know, I know," he laughs at their nonconfession. "They're natural things too, part of human nature, but they can be our own worst enemy. In this passage, Paul tells us to that prayer lets you strengthen your inner man, or woman, I suppose, as a way to *empower* ourselves, a word they throw around a lot these days in SA."

We've heard a few people here share others like it—challenge, corruption.

"If I ask your son or daughter, or some of these sisters or your roommate here, will they tell me you show love to others? Or will they tell me you're a gossip, or angry?"

The response he gets is a few squeaks as a few of the residents shift their weight in their chairs.

"It's hard, I know. I know some of you pray for things like for the All Blacks or Springboks to win, or a Ferrari"—an easy-out to cut the tension—"but I'm also saying this for your health and comfort. So that you'll also pray to strengthen that inner man. Let the gossip go because it will also improve your health. You might not need those drugs back there as much as you think. I'm not saying you don't need them for your cancer or what ails you now. But there's pain in life in a bigger sense. And with prayer, it can be less. God will be impressed."

Remember what Angel said, that when we die, the pain leaves, but life carries on.

I've been wondering what that could mean since she said it. That there's an afterlife where we stay active somehow, unencumbered by that which ails us? What if the pain was due to physical aging? Do we have to keep our same bodies once we get to the other side? It's strange to imagine Heaven being full of mostly older or frail people who died in late life, along with younger ones lost to war, disease, or car accidents. Maybe God lets us choose how old we'll get to be, free of pain.

And God—who is He? What else does He want us to do in meantime, as we wait in this spot a little while longer?

Or should we say "She" for God? There aren't gendered pronouns in most of the black African languages spoken around here anyway.

Intro to Women's and Gender Studies, or even the most basic course on feminism, would show you that that gender isn't about studying women only or that men are inherently bad. It's about studying power. It's just that when you look at who has power in a real, has-an-effect-on-your-everyday-life kind of way—who tells you what to do, makes the decisions that affect whether you get what you need, or makes decisions about what to call you—it's usually men who have this power. Men in law enforcement, business and politics, health care and churches.

In most of the African languages spoken around here, God goes by other names for men—Lord, King, Nkosi, Father, Baba, Mkulunkulu, the last one combining "grandfather" and "the Great One." Maybe thanks to the way it was translated biblically in the first place by the missionaries. They made us forget that women and others are goddesses too.

Maybe God is more of a "They" or an "Us"—a collective power that wells up from the total sum of us human and more-than-human beings in this world. Human power is godlike in some ways. The laws and protocols we put in place determine the course of someone's life, whether someone lives or dies, when and how. We see this power in a wide range of occupations, from executioners to the those who work here and use more tender tactics—withdrawing care, withholding food, or water, administering particular medications in the end. Giving less than the bare minimum to support life—"comfort measures only," Charlie tells me it's called in U.S. hospice.

I don't mean to make it sound like nurses or any medical provider, of whatever gender, have total control over the fate of their patients or residents. To care is to engage in an unstable relationship where each side must make the effort to mind the other in their respective quest—to heal, be healed, or to know when, in fact, it is the best time to end things.

In my mind, for providers at least, care for others should be guided in part by the knowledge that they themselves will need to be cared for one day, that their own fate will likely lie in the hands of another.

Even with all the talk of a loving God we heard from Father Matt and the others here today, I still somehow picture Him to be more like an all-knowing judge, jury, and executioner.

("And what have you done to deserve entry to the Kingdom of Heaven?" God will ask.)

"I, without qualification, apologise for the pain and the hurt and the indignity and the damage that apartheid has done to black, brown and Indians in South Africa," said the last white president of this country, F. W. de Klerk, in one of his final interviews.[1]

On the day de Klerk died, whiteness studies scholar Christi van der Westhuizen published an article arguing that de Klerk's decision in 1990 to free all anti-apartheid political prisoners, including Mandela, was not based on a "Damascene conversion to the principle of black majority rule."[2] He was just being economically practical as local, white-dominated industries and international investments in the country kept declining—a long, slow downturn.

("Straight to Hell you go," will be His last reply.)

~

At the piano Barra lifts her head to face the ceiling and begins to play the musical closer—what could be the home's anthem—"Amazing Grace." To me, the nineteenth-century hymn is chilling. The rising then falling melody, rising and falling like a wagon wheel trundling over hill and vale. Closing my eyes, when they reach the verse about "10,000 years," the tannies shrink away, becoming starry specks in biblical spacetime, frail bodies "shining" as part of cosmic eternity. It is my mom's favorite hymn.

"Ready?" Bethal asks as she hits the last chord.

Barra bats him off to join Eunice, Jane O. and few others who've formed a little fangirl circle around Father.

Precious, Bethal, and I make off to talk about what we heard.

"My sister encouraged me to pray like that, with force," Precious tells us, "but it didn't feel right to me. She got the idea from one of those fire churches where you pray until you're sore and the pastor throws the fire down on you," making her hand into the shape of an aspirator to pretend-suction something out of Bethal's shoulder. "God pulls out the bad and in-dwells the Holy Spirit. They're rolling on the floor when that happens in the church, and for what?"

"For the power!" says Goodness who just came up behind us. "But those fire churches say they will heal you too."

"Those churches are also all about the money, the get-rich-quick way to pray," laughs Bethal, rubbing his shoulder. "They don't have real power. People there tend to pray for things you could get anywhere, like money or a car. You should just get a job or go to a mall! You don't get it from 'fire.'"

Fire churches are the more-dramatic churches among those my colleagues call "Charismatic Pentecostal," churches that traffic in the prosperity gospel and have been some of the most explosively popular churches around here for the past twenty years. Some say they sacrifice care and community in their spiritual warfare to cast out demons and call in wealth. Ilana van Wyk calls them a "church of strangers."[3]

"Mm," Precious agrees and bucks her sister further, "that kind of prayer's not what God's looking for."

"So what does God want instead?" I poke.

"God wants you to deal with how you treat people, like the pastor said," explains Bethal, "that you're not angry or doing gossip around everyone."

"It shows you're more hung up on everyone around you, when you should be happy you know God," adds Goodness.

"What if they *can't* do that?" I shift to refer to a few of the older adults they're in charge of. "You know, the few around here who are always angry or depressed. They're sort of stuck in a rut. To me, I'd say it's not really their fault"—the ones living with dementia, who Marina or the other nurses would otherwise call "aggressive" when they bicker daily.

Goodness: "It's not. Maybe God knows that they can't pray that way or change."

"But God can fix that, can't He?"

"Well, some of us have to help them," she admits.

GOD 133

"You guys are angels," I say.

They laugh at the role I cast them in.

"Bethal, you told me they do change, or they can, when you help them to learn new things."

"Yes, and there's always gossip, but like I said, I'm not here to entertain, so if you waste my time, you're gone," he replies.

"He's our Somizi!" laughs Precious—the lightning-white-hair-dyed pansexual entertainer-emcee on *South African Idol* and other reality TV series.

"*Voetsek* (F-ck off), he shoots back, giggling. "You do what you can. I'm not going to break my heart over helping someone come to see they must live out their days another way. God's the last to judge us anyway."

"Yes, it's the same as I said too," Goodness reminds us, "some of them can't really change their behavior. They can't control it anymore or overcome what they're dealing with. We just take good care of them. We see it's God's plan for them, even when they don't see for themselves."

They are angels in a sense, knowing and watching these older adults who begin to dis-identify with who they once were, carry the past into the present, and fully dwell in this intermingled meantime—wait, rather, for what I've wanted to know about the most:

What's on the other side of God's waiting room.

"What do you think happens to us when we die?" I ask.

"Well," hazards Precious, "as we say, you 'go home'"—*ekhaya.*

"That means Heaven," says Goodness.

"They all go to Heaven when they die," says Bethal.

"No man, it's not possible," she scoffs.

"How can that be?" Precious adds to the fire.

Seems like they're caught up on the "all," but to me the reaction's a bit much. I try to come to his rescue—"I think we just lose consciousness and life goes out like a candle," I offer.

They all look at me like I'm still talking after my head's been cut off.

"I mean, I grew up learning that some people go to Heaven and others go to Hell," I offer more. I used to believe in the scene of brightly lit, cloud-comforts, columns; I'm now realizing Heaven looked a lot like Zeus's home on Mount Olympus. And I was, for several teenage years, preoccupied with the thought of possibly not making it there anyway, burning instead for eternity for being gay. I went to confession—"reconciliation" as it was renamed by the Vatican—to air my concerns in a small, wood-paneled church room. Whoever was behind the curtain panel told me not to worry and say a few Hail Marys.

"I'll probably go to Hell," I joke, knowing by this point in the tour, they all "know about me"—the open secret I share with Andrew.

"That's probably right," says Precious smilingly in a way that seems devoid of irony.

"But what happens to the spirit?"

"Well, I don't know what happens to the spirit," she continues. "I'll have to Google that one. In our family church we say that we die, but then we're waiting for a Second Coming of Jesus Christ. I don't think the dead will arise again and be walking all over the place. It's more a spiritual one."

Goodness, in contrast: "Look, some people go to Heaven, but sometimes the spirit goes somewhere else. Like it just hangs around someplace even when the person's finished."

"Do they *lahlabantu?*" It's a rite I've seen some folks do around here, sweeping leafy branches around the place of someone's death—a car crash site, a hospital bed—to help them leave the site, be free.

"They can do that thing, but we don't know for sure," concludes Bethal. "We hear about Heaven, but if you die and it's not according to your time according to God, then your spirit will just hang around."

"I bet they know," Precious, jokes, "they're closer to all of this than we are!"

She's referring to two older women who are sitting near us. At the south-facing window, in the sunlight, is Miss Motsa and Mayer, who are apparently wiser to where we go next—Heaven, the ancestral plane, somewhere else close by. Mayer's doing origami of sorts, delicately folding and unfolding facial tissues.

"I dreamt last night," Mayer entices us.

Precious: "About what, tannie?"

Trembling, then: "That, that we are already in Heaven. When I dream, I dream of beautiful, beautiful things like the sky, the moon. The stars above us. We are already in Heaven. The dream shows me this, and that God has a plan for us, so we must go by His wishes."

"Serene," I respond to the nocturnal scene she's painted.

"What do you think, gogo? Where do we go after we die?" Precious asks Miss Motsa, the other octogenarian woman. She adjusts the woman's white knit hat to sit more snugly around her wrinkled forehead, strokes her forearm gently.

Waving her hand toward the nurse's voice, the blind Miss Motsa tells us in siSwati, "God chooses everyone. But a spirit can become a spook that moves around here and there, in the woods or the mountains."

Like Paul Kruger or LaRoux's dream lover with the gold coins, I remember.

"The body is in the ground and there are ancestors down there," Motsa continues, "but there are spooks everywhere, the ones who have no place, did not make it to where they were supposed to go. Sobhuza and the other *emakosi* (spirits of chiefs and kings), the Great Ones are all around us too."

To sum up these beliefs in the afterlife: our bodies are buried where our forefathers, foremothers, and others are too, sometimes at one's own home, as it's long been the norm to have your family cemetery in your home's yard. Like Granda Malopa's family still buried out front by Grace's gate.

If, however, you die somehow not according to plan, God's or otherwise, you're on roaming, unable to rest "at home" or make it to Heaven. Those larger than family

GOD   135

figures also persist as spiritual forces in their former lands, the Great Ones, those big, thinking-themselves-to-be-godlike men like Sobhuza I, and then Sobhuza II, the Paramount Chief and then King of Swaziland (1899–1982), other emakosi, according to Miss Motsa. It's a deep history.

"I wonder then, if *their* spirits are still here," I ponder.

All together looking out the window far down the south lawn, we all know who I'm referring to in asking this. Even Miss Motsa, who can't see, is facing this view of the Malopa family cemetery near the gate.

In the stillness in the afternoon sun, I feel the coworkers collect their thoughts in the quiet moment.

Miss Motsa swallows, then says clearly, "*Mabhalane.*"

In an instant, we look at her and then down toward the cemetery site in the yard—we're stunned. How the blind woman knew it was suddenly there, no one can say:

Mabhalane, a huge white secretary bird—*Sagittarius serpentarius*. It's a berserk menace of a creature, towering at four feet, it's red feathered face looking like it's been slapped amid stark black plumage. Scientists have measured that each pummeling of its long, long legs projects nearly twenty kilograms (forty pounds) of force. The secretary bird gets its second Latin name, serpentarius, because its main target to kill are snakes.

It stomps around the site on its spindly legs, doing a choppy wardance. We're too far to see if it's stomped any slithering prey.

I'm astonished. The coworkers now seem indifferent.

"Their spirits *are* there, Casey," Precious prophesies, "if you believe they are."

I believe that even if I chose *not* to believe in such things, the spirits of the buried community members would still be there regardless—wandering, as spooks or in some other body or form of their previous selves.

"After the case, things did not go the way Grandpa wanted," explains Bethal. Reading the papers in Angel's office earlier, I did see that two judges in two different courts—one regional, one municipal—had deliberated on the land claim matter. They effectively ruled in Grace's favor.

"But there was a ceremony," adds Precious. "The lawyers from the mother office came, the management, and others, and they had talks with Grandpa Malopa and the committee. Angel and Noeline helped to organize things. I do trust Sister Zaayman the most on these things," she goes on, "to do something right."

Bethal: "Me too"; and Goodness: "And me."

"It was before they finished building the last cottages down there. After the court thing was over, they let Malopa and the family bring a sangoma. They all left her alone for hours down there at the site. When it was over, she came to them, to Angel and the lawyers, and said they mustn't build there and there, where the grass is still bare," pointing down to where we saw the big white bird, now gone. "They agreed, and they put the matter to rest."

An accommodation, or something like it, for more than half a century of legal-but-unethical occupation of someplace that was never supposed to belong to them, as Antjie Krog wrote.[4]

"I do think they can be a good organization," Bethal admits of Grace's mother office,

"Sometimes."

~

Marina passes by with a younger white woman. Another tour's come to an end.

She's in her early forties, cascading dark curls, black leather jacket, jeans—not skinny ones, obviously—she's old enough to know what's fashionably out and in. That thick air of someone who did a few years in Brooklyn after college, was an agent, or had one, brings friends to the continent to have a *jol* (good time) of a week-end at the Park—*verklempt*, bereft.

"There was a time when daddy and mommy took care of each other. Now mommy cannot take care of daddy anymore. That's where we do it for you. But I did say we are now full, shame. But you get the picture now of what we do, how he can enjoy his time here," Marina empathizes, explaining the situation to the now-tearful woman as if the woman were a young child.

Goodness grabs a piece from Mayer's little origami tissue art for her. She daubs her cheeks.

"In-take depends on God's plan. We just wait and see who goes where. Some move back down to their cottage if they get better. Some go home with the kids. Just last month one went home after being here a year and a half."

That was a man named Cobus—"Thank God," Noeline and Precious had said when he left—he was always unwilling to eat, "naughty" for swearing at the staff and masturbating in the bathroom.

"Some in C wing—independent-living—go down to the Alzheimer's, so there's a lot of moving around," Marina says to offer her hope. "Space frees up. You just wait."

Her wet choke means, "Yes."

"God is great. I see His plan here every day."

Mama Zulu

Those after-three-o'clock feelings are setting in—the time you need a pick-me-up or second wind to finish the shift. Something to drink maybe—they just served us tea, but maybe something stronger? An iced coffee (not a thing here), or iced tea? A margarita? I do love a sundowner.

Maybe you wouldn't know what *else* that term means unless you've had a loved one with dementia or you've treated a loved one like this. I learned it from Charlie. Late afternoons, when the sun starts to wane back toward the horizon, is a time when some people living with dementia start to get more active— "confusion, aggression, ignoring directions, pacing, wandering" are part of the symptom cluster sometimes called "sundowning," explains one Mayo Clinic doctor.[1]

Maybe it *is* more like the aftermath of a happy hour.

"They will start to perform for us now!" Precious laughs.

Around the table in the A wing sitting room, a few of the residents are a bit hyped up from their tea with heaps of sugar—story time and few more jokes are on the horizon.

"*Hamban' langaphand'*" (Everyone outside), she commands. Last year, a construction firm donated a green metal canopy and concrete patio with a few foldable card tables, just beyond where Angel had parked the bus. It's a nice to spot to sit and talk, like she said.

A whole crew gets to escape this place, temporarily at least—Precious unlocks the patio doors for Mama Zulu, Miss Motsa, Little Marie, wheeled by their caregivers Goodness, Bethal, and Yolanda. I get to wheel "MaZulu" as they call her sometimes—Jane Zulu, a mother, mama, hence the "ma."

Like the woman who sold me the nuts this morning, I guess we go with "mama" instead of calling her "gogo," even if Jane could clearly be a grandmother. Again, more honorable ways of doing things.

138   GOD'S WAITING ROOM

In this crew, we whites are in the minority—Little Marie and me. Mama Zulu and Motsa, along with Mr. Xitangu in his room, usually play that role as the few black residents in Grace's bigger mostly white family portrait.

Like we learned this morning from Angel—for her at least—integration in South Africa today can mean a few things: that older people across the racial, class, and care-needs spectrum can live together in a place like Grace because each pays as they can, with a little helping hand. It can mean that whatever your race, language, gender, sex, ability, age, and how these intersect with your ability to pay, you are a part of something bigger that is both complicated and ideally communal. Integration can mean that as part of something bigger—the home itself, the nation, some sort of humanity—you should be, on paper at least, free from discrimination. It can mean that in a place like Grace, you can choose to sit, chat, and eat together with others who are unlike you.

Or not.

We know there are criticisms of integration as policy and ideal. That integration policies may be founded in part on problematic assumptions about black and other people of color and shaped by white saviorism and institutionalism.[2] That to institutions first built by and for whites, like Grace, black people and other people of color will never fully belong, no matter the degree of integration. And that Equity, Inclusion, and other lofty initiatives—not totally unlike like our Diversity training this morning—are sometimes just integration by other names. That they will never work to transform such institutions—that a focus on integration obscures communities of color's ongoing oppression and underdevelopment.

Integration can obscure needs for justice and reparation based in material conditions like restitution, as well as utopian possibilities of separatism by and for people of color. Alternative institutions or formations, by and for people of color—in the United States or South Africa, like historically and still majority-black colleges and universities—where people can thrive. Otherwise places and worlds.[3]

We have to make these criticisms, because I'm not sure that integration means it's all sunshine and rainbows as Angel thinks, or we used to hope it would be, either here or there.

~

On the road trip, before stopping here, I heard a few other white supply-side perspectives on how different people could "integrate" in places like Grace:

Tom and Lorraine, directors at a more upmarket old age home.

"Where is your market headed?" I'd asked this married couple.

Tom: "There are too many private frail cares in the area. There are some public ones, run by the women's association, like Autumn Acorns."

MAMA ZULU 139

That association—the SAVF, the Suid-Afrikaanse Vroue Federasie or South African Women's Federation—was one of several similar groups that emerged in the early twentieth century after their white communities' loss to the British in the Second Anglo-Boer War. They focused on white families' social welfare, especially the "poor" among them, and they continue their transformative charitable work today across the country. In its beginnings, SAVF was not as radically white nationalist as some others, wrote the journalist Charl Blignaut.[4]

"There's also Grace up the road," added Lorraine.

"What's the public-private difference?" I'd asked them.

"Cost," said Tom. "There are very few blacks who use private care as most are destitute, so we usually get mostly white clients. The public ones get a few SA beds"—again, beds totally subsidized by the government—"but we don't do that. We've very, very few black clients, maybe one, some time ago. Her medical aid paid for it. She was wasting to nothing from HIV, so it paid for her stay here."

"It's about the money," Lorraine affirmed.

And Tom: "The black market is huge potential. In that population, the people look after their old ones, but frail care for them will be for the growing middle class. When a black man becomes middle-class, he wants a nice car and clothes. Once he affords those things, it's a start. Most cannot afford to send their old people to frail care yet. But as more start to do so, the market will be huge."

"There's just no money in it still," Lorraine repeated, like a cuckoo.

At least in the congregate-living, pay to rent-the-room-and-care-service kind of model. Private properties with levies, like Grace's independent-living cottage model, are more lucrative.

"You should go see them there. I'll call the manager and tell her you're coming," Tom offered.

Two others I met said something similar—white women realtors, Martie and Elsabie, at a welcome and marketing office for a new suburban subdivision. The subdivision was still under construction but would include a "maturity village," frail care, and chapel, among hundreds of non-age-specific residential plots and a clubhouse. Its main anchor: a new private hospital. Everything was branded orange and bright avocado green and named after an indigenous tree—the kiaat.

The realtors told me the land was donated by a pharmacist-turned-farmer who wanted the hospital built first. Some of the hospital administrators or upper-level staff could invest and build earlier on, he envisioned. The rest of the market would follow.

After living for more than a year in a private development like this, South African anthropologist Renugan Raidoo wryly characterizes such places and their investors as anesthetizing an unequal reality by making it prettily "inoffensive" so that everyone in the market is enticed to buy in to it. A place like this might embody crucial things we aspire for—a sense of independence for ourselves or older adults in our lives, security, good infrastructure, health care, and landscaping—yet also feel alienating or contradict our political principles in that environmental degradation and economic inequalities are often perpetuated by places like this. In short, all these contradictions might make us cringe.[5]

So, who will invest first?

"Lots of people around here. This city's outgrowing itself and the townships around it too. African culture says you must take care of old people in their homes," said Martie, "but blacks bought a few of our first plots in the maturity village! Four I think!"

"I made the sales," Elsabie eases in with a tone that's greater-than-thou.

"OK," Martie smirks, "but our boss was really surprised. We were happy to see it because it's not affordable for many. But they're getting more money and becoming middle-class. As the black market grows, it is going to be huge."

(Of course, in the United States at least, we know that the foundations of contemporary real estate practice were built by way of racist policies and practices.[6])

And of course, people who are supposedly part of this new market have their own perspectives.

In a squat yellow book called *Black Tax: Burden or Ubuntu?*, the writer Niq Mhlongo and some of his fellow middle-class or middle-class-aspirant black South Africans share life stories about themselves, their family members, and their communities. These movers and shakers speak to an array of social obligations and life processes made ever-more challenging by the gross financialization of everyday life in the country.

In the past two to three postapartheid decades, young professionals like themselves have come of age through an improving secondary and postsecondary education sector and made their way into entry-level wage-labor gigs. Many find themselves simultaneously supported and compromised on this proverbial path to success by family members who never had such chances. Out of this contemporary socioeconomic morass, and of course due to the country's history, most young professionals characterize their position as something negative, both in pop culture and their personal experiences. Black tax—to pay, loan, gift, and help out family members close and extended who see you as a lifeline—is a social dynamic layering aspiration and anguish.

Some of Mhlongo's colleagues also talk about old age homes like Grace in a theoretical sense, a "what if" possibility for their elders in this new middle-class field.

Phehello Mofokeng recounts how he shared a home with his 106-year-old great-grandmother up until she died, their living arrangement an effectively mutual and intergenerational payment on the black tax. His great-grandmother raised Mofokeng's father after Mofokeng's grandmother remarried and left him utterly destitute, and Mofokeng came to live with them too. "Today," Mofokeng writes, "many grandparents and great grandparents are confined to unloving, sterile and foreign old-age homes—just so their children can live in comfort and luxury. If you view taking care of your parents as any form of taxation, then you will find nothing wrong in sending them to an old-age home."[7] Mofokeng describes how he also later built home for his father, as an act preventing him from going to an old age home, and as a place to bury the umbilical cords of his children.

Also in the book, the writer Sukoluhle Nyathi explains the reality that some young adults have had to defer their own dreams first to build something substantial for their parents and siblings, to make a comparative point that it would also be unconscionable to nicely house yourself before your elders: "How can you live in a mansion when your parents live in a shack?"[8] Or an old age home, maybe.

In Ghana, for comparison, younger and middle-class black professionals lodge similar criticisms about old age homes, be they foreign or unloving. Older adults themselves, however, do not mind them or experiment with alternative living and caregiving arrangements to get by and feel like less of a burden to others.[9]

Here though, in multiracial South Africa, black families' negotiation of this anticipated dilemma is also comparatively worse than whites', Nyathi writes, given the latter's "generational wealth" and that caregiving in white households was long afforded by black domestic workers. Not unlike some of those characters in the book recommendations I first gave you, perhaps—Coetzee's Florence and Mrs. Curren, Higginson's Beauty and Patricia—or here, Andrew's family and Maria, or anyone else really.

Still, because of "class," "culture," and many other reasons, it is true that old age homes are not really that common yet for black families to use. HAALSI might show this.

HAALSI stands for "Health and Aging in Africa: A Longitudinal Study of an INDEPTH Community in South Africa." It is a huge project embedded in a population health and sociodemographic surveillance program that's been going on since 1992 in a nearby district of communities called Agincourt. They do wide-ranging surveys and assessments related to the health and socioeconomic status of householders across the life course. It takes place in communities where Bethal, Goodness, and much of Grace's black staff comes from.

The HAALSI team's research protocols and findings are mostly overseen and analyzed by white researchers, both South African and non-, from educational-institutional places like Wits, Stanford, Heidelberg, Harvard. The actual data collection of canvassing over five thousand black older adults—individuals over the age of forty—in "the field" is done by black researchers.

They've monitored, evaluated, and measured everything from the way receiving an old age grant correlates to low blood pressure, to how much sodium "deprived" older adults excrete via urine spot samples, to general depression and social isolation, to factors that will show that someone is more likely to be uncared for in their home when living with dementia. In total, the HAALSI team has put out probably more than a hundred academic publications about what it's like to be old in South Africa.[10]

None of them focus on black older adults in long-term care settings like Grace, however.

~

I wonder what Mama Zulu thinks of it in here.

It'll be best to hear from her rather than her black peers. Mr. Xitangu doesn't talk anymore, nor leave his room where they play him reruns of the 1970s show about an old-time train passing through the Karoo. He clutches his blanket to his chin when Precious closely shaves him and jokes that she is his girlfriend. The scent of cedar lingers—the scent of his aftershave balm, a wooden cross hanging above his gurney. Miss Motsa has things to say, gets out of her room to sit and eat, but she tires quickly of talking and chokes a lot.

"Child, there is no problem I see in here," Mama Zulu begins, sharing with me in siSwati.

"Life is good?"

"Eh, life is good. It is a good because God is here, and I believe!"

Precious: "Hey Zulu! She's preaching now!"

"She's from around here," adds Goodness, "another homegirl!" Bethal laughs—everyone is going to help Mama Zulu tell her story apparently—recalling that she's ninety-four years old. Born 1929, 1930, or 1931, they guess. Age is sometimes a number that people cannot remember.

"I was an orphan when I was small," Mama Zulu continues. "Mother and father died when I was small, small. My people told me, 'They were sick and died.' I went on living with them, and then I remember I went to stay with small father on the farm"—"small father" (*baba'ncane*) means her father's younger brother. "They were farming in Lekazi," setting us in place and time.

Many nearby places bear the name Lekazi, like hospitals, schools, and shops. It is the old name for the current large township of KaNyamazane, meaning "where the antelope are." Lekazi was part of a larger settlement called Nsikazi, which, in the early twentieth century, was established as a "native reserve" area near the whites-only Nelspruit metropolitan area. It is where black communities came to live as they were pushed farther out from what became Kruger National Park, from other lands that were given to whites to farm, and from increasingly expanding and segregating towns.

Nsikazi was where Grandpa Malopa and the other families were sent to from here, from where they once lived. On the land that became Grace and where their ancestors still lay. In 1962, the apartheid state delegated that Nsikazi should be semi-self-governing under the Black Authorities Act with six "tribal authorities" (the state's terms, not the people's), one being the Mdluli Authority: Goodness's surname.

And eventually, in 1972, the apartheid state linked Nsikazi and two other reservation areas of Mswati and Nkomazi that weren't even geographically contiguous into one giant "homeland" called KaNgwane for people they categorized as tribally Swazi[11]—a racial-political gerrymandering. Since at least the nineteenth century, the area was dominated by clan groups like the Mdlulis, who'd separated from the Dlamini polity, which ruled lands known today as the Kingdom of eSwatini. The Mdlulis now run a luxury safari encampment just within Kruger Park's borders—Charlie and I vacationed there once—a successful land claim. Not everyone in the area identified as Mdluli though. They included people who identified as Nhlanganu and Zulu: Jane's surname.[12]

"My grandmother was the one who raised me. She stayed with baba'ncane. She was strong!"

"Our gogos had to be," Goodness says, adding more context: "Their husbands had to run away back then to work in the mines"—gold, diamonds.

"She made me run too!" Jane squawks, "always up and down to find their cattle. That was *too much!*" (*kakhuuuuulu*).

"What was it like back then?" is my next, again too-open-ended question.

"As a young woman, they said I was too sick. I did not feel like I was dying. But my gogo had a vision that something was wrong with me," emphasizing that, in her family's vision at least, she was truly in bad shape. "Baba'ncane said there was a problem with my legs and feet. That I did not grow. I don't know what that was."

Malnutrition, maybe.

"It did not rain for many, many months. So, my gogo said, 'No, something must happen.' So she sent me to train"—*kutfwasa*, the training to become a sangoma.

"Where did you go for that?" asks Yolanda, breaking her silence among the colleagues with an intent curiosity.

"This one is like Zulu," Precious rolls her eyes to her young caregiver colleague asking the question.

How so, I briefly wonder, and then see that Yolanda the caregiver is wearing a bracelet of white and red beads. They're not part of the standard uniform for her rank at Grace but tells us she's a healer of another kind:

Like Mama Zulu, Yolanda is also a sangoma.

Two diviners of two generations in the same old age home.

I wouldn't have gambled on those odds.

"She wants to know about your training school, where you took your certificate exams!" Goodness encourages Mama Zulu, laughing in recalling her own degree program journey and the joke that, of course, one does not take certification exams to become a sangoma.

Sangoma "school" or training is organized as a few students under the apprenticeship of someone honorable, wiser, and older, a teacher who's undertaken the journey to become a medium themselves so as to heal others. The impetus for taking this learning journey yourself is that you've had a calling—the voice within or on the other side is often a voice of a generations-long-deceased relative you've loved or never known encouraging you to do so. Sometimes, the calling manifests as an illness that fails to heal or a more unnamable feeling. It will never go away, or will only be ameliorated, if you go.

"It was in the mountains," says Jane.

"Where else would it be?" laughs Precious.

"What happened?" I ask her to elaborate.

"My grandmother found a boy who said he would take me there. That boy was a dog! I'm telling you! A thief! Along the way, always pushing me to lie together when we stopped—to find drinking water, rest all day, what what."

"The bastard," laughs Bethal.

"That happens a lot, I heard," scoffs Goodness. "There are false sangomas everywhere!"

Yolanda mews, "That did not happen for me."

"There was nothing that boy had to do with the training," Jane yelps, "or to look out for us who went there. He made me want to run away from that whole training thing!"

"You should have run away, gogo, you can't trust them. They are too much" laughs Precious, whose tone suggests she's *not* amused or convinced by the whole sangoma "lifestyle" or their powers.

Jane: "Kakhuuuuulu! "I had never seen such a place before or things like that. Who knew what would befall me, yoh! They made us stay together in the roundhouse. Five of us!"

The word she uses for the house literally translates "to kneel and pray" (*sigcukathandaz'*), to convey the way you enter the grass-thatched beehive structure, bent down nearly crawling on your knees to pass through the small door—it is always dark inside, where ancestors are. It's best commune with them in these shrouded surrounds.

"You learn so much there," says Yolanda, speaking from her own training experience. "You learn about your dreams, what you must do and not do if you see things around you.

"Like what?" Bethal questions.

"In a dream, when you see a cattle, they are your ancestors," Yolanda instructs.

"That one we know," states Goodness about the apparently obvious.

"Snakes also. Black, yes. White, yes," the young sangoma-caregiver explains further, charting the more than symbolic associations, "but not green ones. If a green one passes you by, you should seek more answers from us about what it could mean."

The other caregivers murmur—best not to pass up anything new you might learn about things that are outside your purview.

"You must pass by it, not engage with it," says Precious, trying to end this topic.

"How do you know that?" asks Bethal, to which Precious doesn't answer. She asks Jane: "Ma, what did you learn?"

"Yoh, many things. I saw the ones underground"—*labaphansi*, the buried ones, the dead—"They called to me. It was for many moons. I listened and I knew things," Mama Zulu says, not so gravely.

We're silent now, the staff and I, Miss Motsa. Little Marie is at the other end of the card table, humming to herself—a folk song about wandering.

"Then I went back home to the farm, to baba'ncane. But I say to you now, when I got home, this happened: *all of it* was lost."

"Shewww," the staff exhale together, taking in the climax.

Meaning what? I fidget, not getting it.

"It"—her chronic affliction, calling, the ancestral plane now embodied and channeled into a healer's life through training. "It did not follow her. It all just leaves you sometimes," Yolanda explains.

"I thought that it *will* follow you, even *if* you don't use it," states Goodness, a more dire prospect.

"God loved me!" Jane interjects. "He saved me from it! I don't know why. I just went home, and it never followed me there. My gogo was not concerned. I was not disturbed by it either way. This is what happens," she concludes. Maybe her experience is a caveat to what we learned about lost souls—the deceased who die before their time, who roam away from home like wandering stones. Maybe the dead do not haunt or follow us wherever we go.

"Zulu, were you married?"—*kushada* is the term Precious uses to pivot topics, the general term for marrying but more for a white wedding in church with banns and a white dress.

"I was never married!"—in the kushada way, at least. "For that, we had nothing. Baba'ncane found a man for me, and they arranged it. And then the man was my husband. They paid my lobola, but hieeeeee . . ." she squeals.

She knows the caregivers are waiting to hear how much her husband's family paid for her lobola, the bridewealth amount they organized and gifted to her family. It should usually be several healthy cattle, for the wedding feast and for Jane Zulu's brothers to keep and save for their own lobola needs for their own future wives' families, respectively. Jane's big reveal:

"It was 7 rand!"

The staff howl. It is laughably pitiful. "And no cows?" squeals Precious.

"Girls, just think of the inflation," I say. Don't embarrass her—the oldest inflation calculator I can find online would make that around 700 rand today, about $40. It was likely only money, too, not cattle, due to black families' increasingly insecure land tenure in those years.

"I did not suffer! It was good! I was your age," she says, patting Yolanda's arm, so somewhere in her mid-twenties in the early 1950s. "Then my parents died," this time, baba'ncane and his wife, "so I stayed on by my husband's people. I have three children, only one is late"—deceased. "Sindisiwe (Alvira), Siphesihle (Ellinah), Siphokazi (Dinah)."

She uses the present tense for these relations—"I have." Her counterpoint to my previous thought—the dead are never really gone from our lives.

"And my husband is also late," gone to Johannesburg for months, a former watchman. ("Not John, but Makhubalo," the name I hear echoing somehow, from a poem.[13])

"God put me on the right way to guide me to what I would do in this life," Jane cedes.

"Amen, Zulu," Precious encourages her, siding with Jane's Christian convictions over the sangoma chapter of her life. It's a definite slight to her sangoma coworker, Yolanda. Yolanda doesn't seem fazed.

146   GOD'S WAITING ROOM

"When my husband died, I was also sick. I was so tired every day. For work, my brother went to crush the rocks at Witbank," some mine or quarry. "He went to Watchtower"—the Jehovah's Witnesses. "My brother said to me, 'Come.' So I went. I decided to go to him from where we were staying at Lekazi."

By that time, the 1980s, Lekazi and other places here had become dangerous. There was anger in these communities that welled among young people like the Comrades whom Goodness fought for. Anger at those who continued to support the white-appointed homeland administrators, the majority-white police, and those black men who became double agents and assassins for them, like the Kabasa gang—"their job was to kill young black people"[14]—people like Zulu's daughters, Goodness, and other young black people who protested then for change.

"At Watchtower, I was baptized," Jane says triumphantly. "Who will ask me now, 'Who healed you?' I will say, it was the Great One" (Mkulunkulu)—another name for God sometimes.

Precious, again: "Amen!" Goodness laughs.

"And since I was baptized, yoh! I have never had pain in my life. Before then, I would go to the clinic all the time, I was so sick always, even as a young person. And now, until this day, I only take Panado"—paracetamol, for general aches and pains.

And so it goes, her life story shaped nicely and tightly into before and after, dark to the light, ill to well. It's an easy and also patently Christian way of narrating one's journey on the road to anticipated redemption or Heaven.

"Now I only dream of Sister Marina," Jane quips, "she's the one who gives out the pills when my head aches!"

We all laugh at that one.

"Yoh, my children," she sighs, naming the listening staff members among us one by one as if they were her own, "it's a story."

She and Yolanda—the two sangomas—remain entwined in arms. The younger caregiver strokes the older woman's sweatered arm.

"I knew Zulu was a good one. It's why *it* did not follow her," Precious explains. "You don't let that belief come into you, that someone is doing something to you. Even if you have money, and something bad happens, a sangoma or the spirits will tell you it's your sister, your old neighbor who is preventing you from getting married or finding a job or whatever," more cynically reiterating what Goodness told us earlier. "Most people here will believe that. But there is different way of thinking. That if you're poor or suffering, you're not working hard enough."

My first thought goes to the worst stereotypes of "poor" people in the United States, the policies forcing the most vulnerable to work for bare-bones assistance. Fortune tellers or psychics you might consult will say something similar—you're blocking yourself somehow, you are stuck in your own jealousies or attitudes, or you are hung up on someone else's misbehaviors, rather than the subject of others' malevolence or a general maelstrom that leads you to have more problems than others.

My second thought is that I'm not sure Precious or anyone for that matter can be sure if it's God's plan, or the lingering touch of the ancestors around us—ghosts or spooks—who move us long the road of life to our final judgment and transition. In ways that feel unexpected.

"Bethal, what do you think," I ask—he's been mostly silent, looking a bit muddled by the whole spiritual discussion of whether one has control of their fate or someone else has control.

He bites his lip and gives a less than convincing shrug, "I've just heard stories about these things, so it's what these ladies say, I guess. I don't really know."

"This thing is about *us*, not them," Precious snaps to Bethal, and then to me, "so don't worry Casey, you're safe here!"

About black people's fates, not whites—racial differences on metaphysical level, apparently—that witches or sangomas apparently don't deal with white people, even though I've known a few white sangomas in my time and whites who act like witches in the worst possible sense.

"So none of the people in here are at risk for that?" I ask, referring to the older white residents. Nearby, Little Marie's stopped humming—just gently breathing, eyes closed.

Goodness: "No, man. What else is their problem besides old age? No one is coming for them. They just pass according to God's plan."

I don't think it's that easy. You can be cursed by any one, I hazard. I once heard a colleague liken a cancer diagnosis to a witchcraft revelation, a curse-like diagnostic truth that someone with power like a doctor or healer of any kind invokes upon you at your weakest moment. Revealing what's festering inside you, and putting you on journey to find cures and answers about one's fate—the unknown.

"Well," cedes Precious, "maybe witches can affect these old white people because they are weak anyway. They can't get into fasting like some of the sangomas or prophets ask you to do"—it's a strengthening ritual. "The residents have their strict diets. They need their porridge every day to stay fit. And because of the memory issues, they can forget to pray, which you must always do. But now that I think about it, I'm not sure."

"Those abilities are a gift from God anyway," says Goodness, referring to the powers of a sangoma, or psychics maybe, and an assurance that whatever effects they have on us, it's not coming from a bad place.

"It's true," Yolanda quickens, "I always pray to God first even if I am talking to the others"—ancestors, I imagine her to mean—"I need Him to know what I hear from them makes sense, for me to go further to help the ones who come to see me for it. I do pray every night."

"Me too," quips Precious, "but if I have a glass of whiskey, I forget"—another good sundowner.

"It can seem sometimes like He doesn't answer our prayers," Yolanda slows. "It's challenging. You try hard for something and find at the end you achieve nothing."

"I'm joking," Precious admits, "but you do need to be serious in prayer. If I feel blocked, I'll say, 'God please bear with me,' because remembering to go on living each day is hard."

Sniff, sniff—"Mariejkie, you have to change now," states Bethal.

Precious, the auxiliary nurse, looks at Yolanda, the caregiver-sangoma. Yolanda gets up from sitting with Mama Zulu to wheel Little Marie back inside to be changed. The hierarchy of who helps whom in certain situations is clear.

The others decide its best for all of us to caravan back inside. Above the scraping sound of wheelchairs turning under their body's weight, we hear it:

Click, click, click, click.

Heels—you can tell it's a visitor because residents only wear slippers or sneakers and staff only flat round-tip shoes. The latest nurses' union negotiations say your employer has to provide one pair for you the first year you're on the job and one pair the second—brown-colored.[15]

"Gogo, *sengiyeta*" (I'm coming).

"Zulu, Peggy's here," Goodness announces.

"*Lifa lam'!*" (My inheritance!) Jane sings with joy.

The middle-aged woman, Peggy, has two big bags, one in each hand, and a little boy in jean overalls in tow. They veer right to Jane's room. We can hear cabinet doors opening and closing.

"She's bringing you presents!" jokes Precious.

"Lotion and more nappies," Peggy says, joining us at the sitting-room table now—a private stash for Jane to use with the staff's help. No hugs or kisses, but Jane seems happy the two are here. For the rest of us, she hands out bags of chocolate Amajoya, swirled Werther's Original-type butterscotch candies. They go fast.

Peggy is Jane's daughter, or actually Jane's sister's daughter. Here, all your sister's kids are your kids, though.

"*That* shift," sighs Precious to Peggy, "I don't know how you manage."

"This month, hey—the tourists come and go. They add temporary staff to help make up for it."

Peggy works at one of the lodges near the Park. Again, it's a busy season, Heritage Month, when it's cheaper to get in like we did on the safari. Fourteen-hour shifts made up of checking in the guests, booking outings to the "bush" with contracted rangers and drivers, begging housekeeping to respond lightning-fast to guest demands.

("Please, sweep out the ants, they're revolting!" and other creatures that are too innumerable and indigenous for anyone to ever dream of keeping out or separate from us.)

There are arguably worse jobs there—staying in tents within the Park at night, cutting bushes during the early, early morning and later in the day to prevent wild-

MAMA ZULU

fires. The risk manifests in actual tragic loss. Some who were lost to the fires also came from Grace's staff members' communities.[16]

"Ready, gogo?"

"Casey, go, help her."

Peggy pulls Jane out from the table. The nurses get in formation—Jane's latest farewell tour. Yolanda calls out singingly, *"Simvalelisa!"* (We bid her goodbye!),

Precious and Linda respond singingly, *"Muntu lohambako!"* (This one's leaving!)

"Simvalelisa!"

"Muntu lohambako!"

"Simvalelisa!"

A bunch of real performers. "They're here to entertain," laughs Bethal.

The last "this one's leaving" rings down the hall as we wheel her further. I'm carrying one bag now filled with some of Jane's folded clothes and nappies for a few days' getaway.

"I'm glad they do her washing," says Peggy.

"I'd be too."

"We get to take her home once in a while, on holidays, school break. When there aren't too many activities going on. When people can mind her," her daughter explains. "I often stay on-site at the lodge. Transport is too much to go home for a few hours then back to work."

It's the same problem for the nurses here, too.

"And I can't help my mom like they do here. She can't walk anymore, she can't bathe herself or eat alone, so this is better."

Jane probably hears everything Peggy's saying but is sort of just chatting to herself about something someone else said, some other time.

"Dinah"—Mama Zulu's daughter, the late one—"applied for her and got her in here. She was also working twenty-four hours a day on-site at an orphanage near us, so she also failed to find time to care."

"It was God's plan," I suggest.

She doesn't respond to that one.

"Dinah passed a few months ago and was doing the most for mom. So I'm learning more."

The little boy beat us out in the parking lot first.

Click, click.

This time the car door, the seatbelt. He opens the front passenger door for his gogo, Mama Zulu, and climbs in the back among some mathematics schoolbooks—grade 4. Transferring Jane is the final job for Peggy and me. She's heavy, and best angling the chair toward the car seat in the swing of the open door is a struggle. It does feel like Peggy doesn't quite know how to do the transfer.

You're supposed to encourage the older person to stand, if she can. If she can't propel off the armrests, put your arms under her pits to lift. Buck her knees with yours as they bend. Then, ask her to dance, meaning do slow, small-step pivots until her back is to the door. Ask her, eye to eye, to slowly sit into the car, laying her head forward to miss the door frame on the way in and down. After, you can lift and turn her legs inward.

Like Peggy said, she'll learn. We all should.

With a cough from the exhaust, their little white Toyota creeps down the bricked driveway to Pretty at the gate. The little boy looks back at Grace through the rear window.

Simvalelisa, gogo.

~

Back indoors, a middle-aged black woman in a pink pajama jumpsuit talks with Angel. The woman sits on a bench while Angel stands.

"Yebo, sis," Yolanda and Goodness offer in greeting her while passing by, off to their next task.

"Ninety-eight years! Your gogo is golden, hey?" Angel beams.

The pink lady's enquiring about a spot for her grandmother in Grace.

Angel explains the costs: ". . . and then what the grant or pension will not pay, you, the family, will top up the rest. There are no beds for now, but there is the wait list."

The woman nods. I wonder if the queue to get in here—now with the dark-haired woman's father, the people from Silverdays home now that it's shutting down, others—really goes by first come, first served. How will she triage?

"I am also a nurse," the woman explains eagerly, "but I'm in administration now. It's a good position—transport and housing stipend—but it's not my calling."

Angel, quickly: "Shame, and the Sisters here know it's tough, neh. Most of the salary has to go to the bus or taxi to get to work. It's not fair, I know. Finding work is difficult. Even here we are overstaffed, and some we call when someone goes on leave." And then, pivoting to reply to what she believes might be the woman's next line of questioning, "We can take your CV and your phone number, sweetness. When the Head Sister"—Noeline—"says she needs you, I can hire. We'll call you."

Their *baie dankie*s (thank yous) are mutual.

After she leaves, I ask Angel about the pink lady's gogo's prospects for a room.

"I mean, they come more and more to see if gogo can stay with us. Everyone is welcome, but I also find that for every four to five we let in, two or three will leave us sooner than later."

"How so?"

She chuckles, again seeing I don't get what she believes is obvious—"The family wants to use their pension."

MAMA ZULU

Me: "Is *that* so," letting my tone and raised eyebrows show that it sounds incredulous.

"Well think about it, if they live at home, that is more money than the old person *really* needs. If they stay here, the whole thing goes to paying for their room, food, and care. It all gets eaten up here."

Instead of where, or how, I wonder.

"It's a heartsore," she waxes momentarily, and then, "I always look at the car they use to drive up to visit. If their car is fancy, it just makes me wonder."

Security

"Reverse, *bhuti*" (brother).

I missed the turnoff by a few hundred meters.

Back in Wisconsin, we used to say "whip a shitty" to make a full 180 when you're going the totally wrong direction. I promise by the end of this, despite the stalls, the wandering among stories, the "what the hell are we reading or doing here's," you'll see we took the right one.

The road simply ends a few kilometers from here at a fence erected among scrub brush and sepia-toned flat earth on an endless horizon. On the other side of the fence is the Park, a few granite boulders here and there stacked by the hands of some gods. Around us, a few one-room cinder block buildings—homes-to-be. Some with or without a door, sheet-metal roof, barbed-wire-and-firewood fencing, a lone tree scraping the blue sky.

Among the bits of habitation, we pass one large double-story house with glass sliding doors, balconies, a two-stall garage.

Goodness, excitedly: "Sam Nzima lived there. You know Sam! That's the house the white people paid for."

That's specific, but I can't place the name while trying not to drive the rental into another pothole.

"You know, he took the picture of the kids who got shot by the police," she helps me to remember.

That's also specific, horribly so, but I know exactly what she's talking about.

The picture—Mbuyisa Makhubo, eighteen years old, carrying the lifeless, school-uniformed body of Hector Pieterson, thirteen, and Hector's sister Antoinette Molefi, fifteen, hemmed skirt batting her legs, running alongside Makhubo, pleading with him to tell her where he was taking her brother. Hector was one of the first of somewhere between 170 and 700 children killed by apartheid police in a mass demonstration of 10,000–20,000 people in Soweto, June 16–17, 1976, who protested the government's mandate to make part of the national school curricu-

SECURITY 153

lum for "Bantu," or black students, exclusively in Afrikaans. Only sports, religious studies, and music were to be taught in the students' mother-tongue black African languages.

After, Mbuyisa was harassed by police and fled the country, perhaps part of an ANC cadre. The last his family heard from him was in a letter dated 1978 saying he was in Nigeria and planned to go to Jamaica.[1] Decades later, Antoinette helped to establish a memorial site and museum in honor of Hector for all to behold and remember. Her extended family is still unsettled over the rights to his name and image at the site.[2] She's seventy-two now.

Sam Nzima took the photo of the trio I'm depicting for you. It was quickly published across the globe—in *Time*, the *New York Times*, *World*, for which Sam worked—catalyzing international opposition to the apartheid regime. A BBC retrospective on the impact of the photo was titled *The Day Apartheid Died*. After its publication, Nzima was put under house arrest. He said the picture destroyed his journalism career, and he only regained the rights to the image in 2002. Nzima became a tireless advocate for his community, the one we're driving through now, calling for new schools to be built, potable water, other necessities. He passed away in 2018.

A sign comes into view once we whip the shitty—Hlayisekani Old Age Home. Again, it means "Security" in Shangaan, Goodness's mother tongue—along with the address, municipal registration, phone contact details, and "Visitors Welcome."

Among its cinder-block neighbors, Security is magenta, solidly roofed, a sturdy fence with sliding electronic gate like Grace, a small fortress protecting its occupants from something out here. Maybe animals that escape from the nearby Park—lions, cheetahs,

Other dispossessed beings.

We trundle in as some invisible guard opens for us.

Under a tree, a few children and their mamas sit for lunch: avocado, again the giant bright green ones, boiled white Colocasia tubers called *madzumbula*. The hot, thick, windless air makes greetings with the women almost inaudible. No one's eyes meet the others. The mutual respect, the deference exchanged with each other is stiflingly liturgical to convey simple messages:

"We see you." "We're just visiting." "Thank you."

I'm useless. Goodness interprets. She bides what feels like an eternity of the nearly silent greetings by surveying the ground around us with the toe of her white high-heel. Then:

"Ha!" There,
    And there,
    A number of miniscule, perfectly circular craters made of piled grains of sand,
    At the center of each, a pinpoint, a darkening hole,
    A portal equilibrating between this world and another.

Out of one, a creature emerges, smaller than the size of a pumpkin seed. Its antennae and pincers luminescent, the color of charcoal.

Not alive it seems, not crawling, but somehow ejected from the darkness.

She picks up the bug and holds it close to my face, lying near a phone number she wrote across the palm of her hand with a blue pen.

"You take ten of these, dead ones. You dry them then grind them. It will come out like Grandpa's Powder"—the packet mix you buy at any pharmacy chain here made of aspirin, paracetamol, caffeine—"You put it back in the hole. You wish for it to work the way you want for someone you love. It will cure their epilepsy and mind problems."

Now, the women are actively listening. One breaks the silence to ask how the wishing part works, and how long you need to dry them out.

"They want my witchcraft things," she winks to me.

The women work inside for Security. Sometimes. One's off because she's mourning her mom who passed last month. Others are more like temps. They hang around should the staff or residents inside need anything. It's something to do— wait to help. They only get paid if the Department of Social Development pays Security its quarterly subsidy, something like 120,000 rand (about \$8,000), or the National Lottery or another sponsor comes through with funds. By the looks of a faded sign on the home's side, they once got a donation from Savanna, the boozy cider company. Otherwise, nothing's come in for seven months.

So, for much of year, they are more like volunteers—"by the kindness of their hearts," Goodness adds—sort of like the thousands of community health workers, unpaid, that sustain many householders' health and wellness across this country, regardless of age.[3]

They do remember Goodness's mom who once stayed here. None happen to remember my colleague, Jessica, who also once stayed here to learn more about Security, how it was established, what "good care" looks like in here versus in your average household in the village, and the sort.[4]

"Mom loved you all so much, too," Goodness awws, shoring up their mutual feelings, and, to me: "My mom wanted to come here so badly. She didn't want to be a burden on Dad or anyone. With her soldiers going down, she should've kept going to the hospital.[5] She went when she first got sick, but it was a bad experience. The nurse said they must take her blood and get a drip, and you know she didn't want to hear it!"

"Why's that?"

"It happens that when you catch a witch like we used to in the Comrades, the person doesn't know she's a witch. It's just something that's in your blood that makes you a witch even if you don't know that you are"—sort of a built-in excuse that accused witches might end up accepting in the face of others' consensus. "She didn't want to find out what was in hers! The nurse was rude to her, too, saying, 'If you don't want us to help you, what are you doing here?'"

I wonder what the nurse thought she herself was there to do if not to treat her.

"So, Mom wanted another option. Grace was too far and too expensive. But she heard me talk about this place and said that it sounded better. So, we fought, like I said, and she made us take her. So we did."

"What happened?"

"She loved the nurses here, their care and love, and the food, yes. They bake bread every day and cook nice food. But she likes food as *she* likes it"—not a picky eater, just judicious—"no beans mixed in *pap* (porridge) for her! Just each plain, or pap with sugar. She asked us to bring water for her too. She said it didn't taste good here."

The home is also the only building in the village with running water.

"After a while, she found that her body was not getting better. So, she said, 'Phone my children, I want to go home.'" We brought her back. She lived about two more years. And then she passed."

Her reason echoes in my mind—"her body was not getting better."

Can an old age home be a place to heal, if aging is an illness rather than cultural, psychosocial, and biocellular process—to cure someone of what ails them, rather than be an almost final place to rest?

Like Grace, you cannot pass into the little world of this home until you meet its angel: here, his name is Panic.

It's actually Nyiko, but Panic, a nickname, is what's listed when one of the women shares his contact details with us on her phone. He's a nurse, too, and the manager who built Security a few years ago from the ground up.

A quick phone call to him—"Yebo, bhuti," says Goodness, rather than addressing him as "Mister," clearly seeing he's younger than her by his picture that appears on WhatsApp—"OK, he will meet us here later." Right now, he's at another home nearby that he also built. That one's a daytime center where older adults congregate but go home at the end of the day. Security is long-term care—residential.

"I remember, he came to see Sister Noeline when I first started at Grace," she recalls. "Many nursing students come for their observations to see how you do geriatrics. He asked to see what we were doing and wanted to make a place like it for the people out here. I think he saw the need."

Let's see for ourselves.

Through the gated door—with his permission and Mandi's, the nurse in charge today—to another one of God's waiting rooms.

This one might be different somehow. Maybe we've instead passed through a portal to a different sort of place, on some other gods' sacred grounds—one made by and for a community, in their terms, not whites. A place we might call an Elsewhere, or Otherwise world I've mentioned before.[6] This one's still being built, bit by bit, but where a different kind of care for older adults—no, elders—might be possible,

156 GOD'S WAITING ROOM

Its occupants moving "always toward"[7] that possibility of something better than what we have already, better than what we've inherited.

Let's see for ourselves.

First, the basics, and the differences: The residents of this home called Security are all black. At Grace, they are almost all white. Cost here is 850 rand ($46) per month. At Grace, it's 6,000 ($330) per month. Both do admissions through an application process. You need a medical report and the report about your background written by a social worker. The manager makes the final call for the final roll—fifty-one souls here, forty-six there.

Both have round-the-clock staff; here there are fewer nurses in the sense of professionals holding a titled degree. More nurses at Grace. Both mostly run on government subsidies, donations, and fundraising—here more, there less. Grace has the levies from the independent-living cottages—white capital. Both run on the residents' grants and supplemental savings—here it's mostly grants, fewer at Grace.

At both, residents enjoy homemade meals made by black women who turn donated foodstuffs into nurturance. The nutritional variety is greater at Grace. Still, both tasty. Security's schedule is 6:00 A.M.: *vukani bo* (wake up); 8:00 A.M.: soft porridge; 10:00 A.M.: tea; 12:00 or 1:00 P.M.: lunch; 5:00 P.M.: a small supper; then, past 7:00 P.M., the night staff share one last tidbit—"or some sugar if they have diabetes," adds Mandi. Similar enough.

A difference: in Grace, it's private rooms or rooms shared by pairs along a series of halls laid out more like a maze. In Security, there's a single passage for easier surveillance, with more ward-like, spacious chambers sleeping around fifteen people in each—two rooms for "ambulant females" two for "ambulant males."

Enter Ambulant Female Room 1, dimly lit, aquamarine:

The beds are a mix of cots and gurneys, each their own soft little world of pillows, blankets, and throws for its main inhabitant. Each room has a bathroom in the rear.

"Those are an improvement from when my mom was here," Goodness says. Like Janice did this morning with the Kardex at shift changeover, she and Mandi give us the rundown, each resident's story and conditions consensually interpreted in real-time through the resident's own words and the two women's nursing experience. Most of the residents are also local. They know where they come from. They're from here too.

"The problems most people face are high blood pressure, stroke effects, diabetes, and cancer," Mandi teaches us. "Some are blind. We just can't take the COVID and TB (tuberculosis) ones because we don't have enough isolation rooms. We can't put them in the general wards or everyone will contract."

Most are wearing masks in some manner—on the chin or on the nose mostly.

SECURITY

Mandi makes the first introduction: "This is Eunice, or Sarisa (her Shangaan name)."

"I think she says she was sangoma," I hazard from what I hear her say. The other giveaway is she's wearing a red headscarf, a bracelet of beads, red and white like Yolanda's.

"Yes, she says she trained in Mozambique when she was young," and then, laughing, "She says *it's all over for you*, too, Casey. You're definitely not going back to America!"

Why? I think my passport's still good.

"She says I'm your first wife," Goodness relays to me, "and Mandi is your second wife. She's gonna be your youngest one!"—"youngest" means "last" here. A tough gig.

With a family I lived with in southern eSwatini in the 2010s, we used to watch episodes of the 2000s HBO series *Big Love*. The show starred Bill Paxton, Jeanne Tripplehorn, and Chloë Sevigny and dramatized American Mormon polygyny, from the gendered violence of the compounds to the wives' quibbles and romances. The mother of the family I lived with, Nokwenza, said it was interesting how they all sort of lived together—in South Africa today, many families like this would not—and the youngest wife, Margene, played by Ginnifer Goodwin, cried the most.

"Eunice here says she'll wake up in the morning to do chores for us. You and Mandi just have to cook for her because I'm the first wife and I'm tired of doing that now!"

Eunice-Sarisa gives another line or two about our new marriage plans—Goodness shrieks with laughter, "Hey, I'm not going to say the rest!"—and then interprets her lasting bit of advice: "If you want to stay active, pray to the small gods of your house—your ancestors—save some of your food for your chickens. They will be eager to eat it, and the gods will give you strength for it. The only health problems she is having is a toothache. She says it makes her feel like she's pregnant again!"

What's the mouth-to-womb connection?

"Being pregnant hurts so you want to just lie down and do nothing like when you have a toothache," Mandi explains, "Just the pain of it. The other pain is that her daughter is in Joburg. She only comes around in December."

Next to this other Eunice is another Marie, or Matšeliso, her Sotho name. She has Alzheimer's.

"One minute she says she has four kids, but then she said she had five. The husband is alive, she says, in Joburg."

Next to Marie is another Yvonne, or Welani, her Shangaan name, wearing a pink hat that could've come from the Grace gift shop, and sitting not on the bed but inside a sort of pillow fort on the floor.

"*Goeie more!*" (Good morning!). Yvonne-Welani fires off at me, and "*War gaan hier?*" (Why are you here?). She and Nettie could tag-team me—"*Praat jy Afrikaans nie?*" (You don't speak Afrikaans?).

"That one is mentally disturbed. 'Alzheimer's' I mean, sorry," Goodness apologizes for using the outdated term.

Between the ambulant female and ambulant male rooms is another room with Security's most blessed residents, those who are closest to divinity, radiating the power of gentleness, in whom I think we can see God's image most intimately:

The ICU.

Two beds, one empty, and one with a woman bathed in sunlight. Her face is young—late forties—her body, light, like a once young tree, now like calm lake driftwood, limbs appearing to ascend through the window.

"Is she 'plus'?" asks Goodness—a spin on another outdated term, "HIV positive" (hence a "plus" sign). It is now best to say "living with HIV" or, in this case, AIDS—Mandi nods.

On to Ambulant Male Room 1: brighter, aquamarine.

Mr. Zeze, whose English name is Andrew, is first. He's bright and bedridden. "Days and days go by here," (*kula' 'malanga*) I hear him say, "but it is comfortable."

"He is brilliant," Goodness says proudly, "He says he used to do canvassing in health outreach. He taught sangomas the primary health care basics in Limpopo and Vendaland."

His shining, watching eyes, the slight haze of an emergent cataract reflect back the gaze of everyone who has loved him for his lionheart.

Sister Noeline told me earlier that she had the same kind of job. Her first career after her retirement from prison nursing, in the early 2000s in KwaZulu-Natal, was as an educator or training nurse who did weekend outreach with sangomas and other healers like Eunice-Sarisa here or, at Grace, Mama Zulu and Yolanda. Handing out packets of razors for single use, for example. Some healers washed and reused blades to incise a source on patients' bodies to insert medicines—homestyle intravenous. Or handing out carbon-copy booklets so that healers could record their patients' treatments and share the leaflet copy with the patient to take as a referral to a hospital like G. J. Crokes, where Noeline worked. Healers like Eunice-Sarisa, Mama Zulu, and Yolanda are smart enough to know there are illnesses they themselves cannot cure.

The next one, a man who has a long exchange with Goodness. There are lulls, "shames" said on her part, laughter, a hand outstretched from his walker to take ours momentarily to bid goodbye.

"He was my neighbor. Mr. Thibela"—whose English name is Johnny—"from Bushbuckridge. I didn't know he was admitted here. He passed on condolences about my mom and asked about my father. He told me when Dad came to visit Mom here, my dad saw some of old people shouting and taking their clothes off, and he said to him, 'We have to get you out of here, it's only sick people!'" she laughs. "That's my father for you."

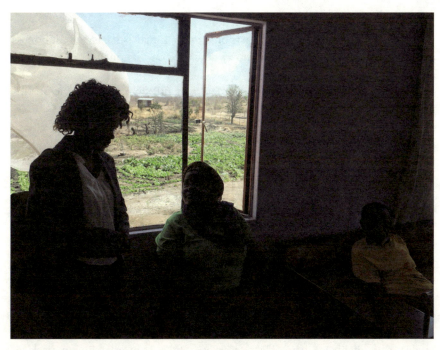

security

"His children brought him here," adds Mandi, "just for his old age, though. He can still walk alright with the Zimmer"—an outdated term for a walker that honors one of its inventors.

"Did they not want to take care of him?"

"It's not a matter of want," Goodness explains curtly. "They were busy working. Some are married. His kids are good kids. They are my age. I know them. One is a nurse in Joburg. I know that one of his kids passed, and when it happened, it was a heartsore. So, they let him come here."

"It's too hard to walk around or go to the bathroom yourself," I say the obvious part out loud.

"Yes, you can't cope," she agrees.

The last room, the main sitting room, their version of Grace's voorkamer with the TV that plays rugby, National Geographic, and opera. Women and men seated, most on pillows or grass mats spread on the tile floor, fewer on individual chairs. Genders separate as if at a church like Goodness's father's. Half don some new green, black, and yellow athleisure wear—jerseys—silky contrasts to the rough cotton flannel, sweats, aprons, and blue workers' uniforms most wear today. "Some more donations," says Mandi, from the ANC, referring to the athleisure wear— "They come sometimes to say they support us."

"We're from eSwatini," Goodness jokes with the women. "We don't get to vote like you, gogos!" Again, eSwatini is a kingdom, an absolute monarchy. You don't get to vote for a king.

160   GOD'S WAITING ROOM

The ladies clap for her little introduction.

A bop-heavy Christian group blasts on a radio. It makes it easy for Goodness and me to try out a few dance-step moves described on a laminated exercise chart affixed to the wall.

Outside the window, a vegetable garden is in full flourish amid the aridity, undulating waves of cabbage leaves suspended in the sun.

One man wearing the political swag comes up tenderly to me.

"*Umfana, ngiyakucela*" (Son, I ask of you, please).

"Yebo, mkhulu."

Five rand, for a cigarette. In my pocket, I *do* have a few coins.

"But don't forget *that*," he says, pointing to my notebook. I left it on an end table.

"*Ngiyabonga*" (Thank you).

"He'll have to go outside. No smoking in here," says Mandi.

Goodness: "He says he used to drive the big tractors around White River, by Plaatjieville. I told him I have the Code 10 license!" That one's for articulated, motor vehicles weighing between 3,500 and 16,000 kilograms (about 4 to 17 tons).

Plaatjieville, I remember, is also where Grandpa Malopa and colleagues made their other land claims, probably on a farm that used those big tractors.

Mandi hands us each another heavy load: lunch—pap, cabbage, a chicken leg—Security's hospitality is memorable for everyone. Still, we can't eat with our mask on.

"Reverse, bhuti!"

~

Back outside in the yard, Panic's already waiting for us. He has his own packed lunch he brought from home. Between bites, the group of elder-care workers talk shop. Goodness breaks down the salary and hourly schedules at Grace, resident-to-nurse ratio, staff numbers, etcetera: "Our 3,500 ($230) per month is basic minimum wage, and even then, after they deduct for our pension, it's 3,200 ($210)."

Mandi says that's racist.

"And at least the staff can live around here," Goodness adds. "The travel is not good, and they don't want to provide for us."

She explains that Angel said that mother office had "protocols" that did not allow the staff to stay overnight within the complex. Most are on a 6:00 A.M.–6:00 P.M. multiday shift. It is an exhausting and expensive roundtrip home, the nasty outcome of the perfected apartheid plan to evict these people far from areas deemed white and yet still needing black labor. Angel eventually converted one room within the main house for staff to stay overnight, but it was in cruddy condition, according to Goodness.

"There were only two twin beds and other nurses ended up sleeping on mattresses on the floor. If you want to go to the toilet, you are stepping around people. It is difficult."

SECURITY 161

Panic says it's probably an occupational or environmental safety concern and violates some other protocol.

"Then they moved us far back to another spot"—inside Grace's complex—"and it was less accessible. So. if there's an emergency with someone in A or B wing, and you must get up to assist the nightshift, you find they are upset when you arrive, saying, 'We've been waiting for you up here to come,'" she scoffs.

Panic: "Apartheid is still here."

And Goodness: "We are not at *emapulaz*'"—siSwati for "farms," from the word in Afrikaans, *plaas*, and meaning they are not to be treated as some sort of beck-and-call laborers—"We are not their maids."

"We serve ourselves here. If there are needs, *I* am the one to make sure we get it," he speaks of Security now.

"What are your biggest needs?" I ask.

"Diapers and medicine. Medicine is not delivered"—at Grace, they get a delivery almost every other day. "I drive to get it, or if someone is sick without it, I drive them to the hospital. People have died in my car on the way."

Again, the heat, windlessness stifles anything except an echo I hear of what happened to Goodness's mother: "Her body was not getting better."

"We're not supposed to be hospice, but it can be. Some people have chronic disease and late-stage cancer. They don't respond to the medications when they have them. So they are just waiting for . . ."

He exhales, and the sentence ends with nothing.

I hasten them to share anything else about this place—"One thing I hear from your colleagues, is that this thing, elder care"—in its institutional sense—"is maybe not part of black culture." I got that sense from talking to Bethal, Precious, and the white providers who said so.

Goodness butts in: "It's not a cultural thing, yes, but the kids want to work or have to put the parents somewhere because they are sick."

"They will do anything for them," I say.

"They get used to it."

"Or they see it's a good thing?"

"Mmm."

And from Panic, another "mmm," And, "It's not really true, that it's not cultural. I think it's something we could have done in the past in another way, but today, people find old age care to be a good thing. I like what we do at Security because we are helping people and making a difference in the community."

"How?" I ask.

"With the Alzheimer's or dementia, I know these are problems for some people in the rural communities"—the intramural criticism, the criticism that many people who are middle-class, whether they are black or white, sometimes make of those they believe to be less educated or blinded by "culture" or "strange" beliefs[8]—"If they see an old man walking around or going to someone's house because they get lost, they end up killing or burning them. I know that. I've seen it."

162 GOD'S WAITING ROOM

Mandi looks at her phone. Goodness watches him, listens. And again, maybe he is saying this to me, this thing about problematic cultures and older adults' insecurity, because I am white.

"So, it is good when they come here. They can be safe or secure. There is no cure for Alzheimer's or dementia, so even if they were home, or here, they would be doing the same. The family might have expectations that we can change that behavior and complain when we can't. They think we aren't doing our job."

("Her body was not getting better.")

"Others here are missing their kids who passed from AIDS a long time ago. They come here through the social worker or the hospital"—at Grace, like Mr. Xitangu and Miss Motsa—"I believe in caring for people who once cared for us."

The debt repaid.

"And because, like she said, the kids who are still alive are working. Like us. Maybe the workplace is very far and they only come back on month's end"—like Mama Zulu's or Eunice-Sarisa's daughter, or the adult children of any white person in Grace—"or maybe they are not working but do not have the skills when someone is bedridden. It is a burden. Like, if an old man is staying with his daughter or the daughter-in-law, and they feel uncomfortable caring for him because he needs a catheter."

I am sure some will tell you they would catheter their parent out of unconditional love. Or because of culture, again—saying no to the obligation would have consequences, the "no" echoing immorally throughout your generations forever. Or because of financial matters—you have to because you cannot afford a home health care worker or someone else to do it.

For those who can afford it—the act embedded in a larger institutional elder care system, where social welfare is also business-like and operates on the backs of working-class women of color mostly—it is still emotionally difficult to even think about it. I am sure there are some critics who will tell you that embodied feeling—shame or abjection maybe, in facing the intimate act of catheterizing their parent—is just another discomfort of being caught within an ageist, ableist, racist system that alienates us from our caregiving obligations.

I am sure.

"They can't take care of themselves anymore, and now it's our turn," Panic concludes, "it's just that before we didn't have enough skills to start facilities like this. If there was money, it was never enough. It *was* only for whites. Not anymore."

Noeline

"*Mr. Mandela is here!*"

Noeline: "That was Matron Pfaff, my boss at Garden City Hospital in Johannesburg, who was shouting about him. She ran straight up to tell me. I remember her eyes all buggered out. And I said to her," blinking unexcitedly, "'So?'"

"'But he is looking for *you!*' she pleaded."

"'So?' I said to her again. 'I looked after that man's health for eleven years on Robben Island. *That* is why he is looking for me.' But Casey, you know, he made everybody crazy when he was alive. So, I said to my colleagues, 'Calm down. Mr. Mandela had a very difficult life, but he is also a human being. And the night he was taken off the island, he promised me that one day, when he rules this country, he will look for me. So Pfaff and I went down the stairs into the emergency department. That's where he saw me and opened his arms. I walked into them and hugged him. He hugged me back and kissed me. You should have seen it. Everyone was looking, and I knew they were thinking, 'Who in the hell is this white lady?'"

Right now, I'm thinking the same.

"Mr. Mandela said to me, in front of all of them, 'I'm happy that Noeline is working for you. Correctional Services lost their best nurse when she left Robben Island. Not only did she care for the health of the people there. She was like our mother in the prison. She was my mother, my psychologist, my nurse, my confidant.'"

A tower of small, upside-down plastic cups shirked from their plastic bag and standing free on the table begins to disassemble in her hands. Looking down from six feet with auburn hair, Noeline moves swiftly, taking one cup from the top to turn upright and drop in white, blue, and orange pills of different shapes. She knows who gets what and reorders them like chess pieces on the cart, saying the names of each recipient and new changes to their regimens. Classes 5 and 6 are habit-forming and stay on the top shelf. She alone holds the pharmacy's key.

A white one falls on the floor. She picks it up and blows on it—a kiss—before putting it in someone's cup.

Louw already wheeled himself over to where we're standing to be first on the afternoon "med pass." He takes a pinky flesh-colored contraption out of his mouth to swallow the pill with a phlegmy cough. Precious comes up from behind and gives him a gold-ring-fingered shoulder rub, then wheels him back to his room. He'll steal away a smoke at his barred window, laughing at something that lies beyond the fence.

Angel passes by on the way to the nurses' station. She's got an armload of red folders—new intakes. Bea, a beautiful blue-eyed woman as they told me, died on Sunday at the age of ninety-four. Her bedroom's opened up for two new people to move in. Word among the nurses is that Maureen, the municipality's black social worker, got Angel to take in two gogos who've been on the admissions waiting list for a year. That would bring up the number of black residents to five out of the near-fifty total souls.

All part of God's plan here. After med pass, we have to clean up Bea's room for their arrival next week.

Noeline's little battlefield of cups is finally ready, laid out on the cart's gauzy blue paper, a thin anchoring for the mostly even-wheeling journey through the hallways. We journey together.

We're on the clock for now, still, but I hazard her time. "I mean, Noeline, working at Garden City, every day you see people come and go. They touch you in a way but leave quickly. They're more like strangers. It's not like here. Or the prison. You see the same folks every day, for a long, *long* time. They're not going anywhere. You get used to them."

The comparison's frail but an easy one to draw, I suppose.

"Casey, *they* get used to *you*, neh. It's not just the other way around," she says.

"Had you done geriatric training with your nursing?"

"I did. And palliative care too. The first training at Sharley Cribb in Port Elizabeth where we would travel every three months by train. I was a farm girl, grew up in the Karoo, and Oudtshoorn was my mother hospital. We went to Cribb for theory, and we traveled to do our specialties. Tygerberg in Cape Town to do midwifery and Karl Bremer Hospital to do geriatrics and palliative care. I went like that for four years."

Cribb is named for a nurses' union leader and reformer whose work led to the creation of the South African Nursing Council; Bremer for a Minister of Health who advanced "separate-but-equal" medical education for "non-Europeans" in the first years of apartheid.[1]

I'm amazed actually at the number of schools she went through to complete the course. "I guess it's helpful to see how people in different places do different things."

"It is," she asserts. "It forms you, gives you information, and a sense of how to handle different people and situations." Her gold wedding ring slides along the rim of a pill cup for Sarie—just one white disc inside for blood pressure.

"And you met your husband in those years, right?" I've heard side-bits of gossip about the love of her life from others throughout the tour, the man she fondly called Rickus.

"In Oudtshoorn, yes. And I was very young when I started nursing. Just eighteen and just out of school. And he was working for the police. We Afrikaners of those days, on the farms, we were brought up very strict. Very strict. You don't go out with men before you're out of school, so my father told me. So, I was extremely naive, and I was afraid. But he also grew up on a farm there, so he was also very naive."

I laugh at her recalling her Karoo valley farm-girl unworldliness, a scene of two teenage-to-twenty-something lovers, awkward with each other and the ropes of their first real-world jobs—policing and nursing—again, both bloody ordeals.

"One night I was working in casualty, where they brought in accidents, and Rickus brought in a man who was badly hurt. When the patient was stabilized and prepped for the theater, he asked me, 'What's your name?' And I told him, 'It's Noeline.' He became my first and last boyfriend."

One and done.

"So we grew together. We went out for six years before we got married. My father"—a postmaster and Freemason—"just said, 'You must first learn, and then you get married, because if you get married right away, you won't have time to learn about each other.'"

"So, it was a test run?"

"Ja, and Rickus was also studying, you know, criminology and the things like that. That's why he also had a very good relationship with the prisoners because he had the training to be good with them."

Rickus quit the Oudtshoorn police and moved to Paarl, a deeply Afrikaner and wine-rich city north of Cape Town, to start a post with the state's Correctional Services unit in 1970. For three years, the two did a long-distance relationship until she finished her training and moved to join him.

"Right," she recalls, wheeling now down B wing, "and I remember I was doing night duty at the time, so I was sleeping during the day. And I heard a knock on the flat door, neh."

Rapt suspicion at the sound is what I take away from the look she gives me.

"I put on my nightgown and went to the door. This man had the same uniform as my husband, but his had all of this braiding and medals hanging from it here and here," she compares, brushing from chest to shoulder and her own epaulettes and enamel pins that show off her superior ranking to the other Sisters working here.

"And being very innocent—I didn't know—I said, 'Hello, uncle, can I help you? I'm sleeping now so sorry for my pajamas.'"

"'Are you Zaayman's wife?' he asked."

"I said, 'Yes.'"

"'How would you like to go to Robben Island?'"

The deadpan delivery of his demeanor—was that really his question? Or a threat? For her, the answer to it was certainly impractical.

166   GOD'S WAITING ROOM

"'Are you crazy?' I asked. 'How is my furniture going to get to there?'"

"'I'll organize a trip for you,' he said. 'Go, decide, and I'll come back to you. The president must give you authorization'"—if it was the South African President who authorized it, it was J. J. Fouche then. "And you know what? We did it. I remember the days ahead, getting ready and walking around the quay in Cape Town. I went up to one of the wardens who was wearing the same uniform as my husband, and I said to him"—in the girlish voice she'd used to greet uncle officer—"'Please tell me, where's the boat that goes to Robben Island?' And he says, 'There she is, the *Suzan Kruger.*'"

Named after the wife of the notorious Minister of Prison Services, Jimmy Kruger, the "*Suzie*" was built as a pleasure cruiser with a lounge, bar, and other "holiday features" in 1959 and bought for what would today be more than $16 million from a German company.[2] Before *Suzie*, she was called the *White Lady* and was the main mode to transport prisoners and staff to the island. In an interview for the Robben Island Museum and UNESCO World Heritage Centre, one former prisoner, Mr. Madlavu, recounted:

"As we entered the boat we were kept below the deck. . . . The travelling on the boat itself to the Island was historical in the sense that I had never been on the sea before. It tended to make some of us want to vomit and we felt that we were now being cut off from society and we would never come back. Never see our families and our friends and I remember one of my co-accused mentioning that when we return we should not expect to see our parents alive. . . . It was as if an umbilical cord was being cut."[3]

Noeline's furniture, the harbor wardens told her, would go below deck on another boat.[4]

The steely med cart brings us into Jane B.'s room, in B wing, to release to her, like Louw, a single blood pressure pill. Last month Jane's daughter Mona hung a gold fleur-de-lis frame with a picture of herself, Jane, and two small children at a beach—Eastern Cape. All together, kneeling in the sand, faces lined cheek to cheek, squinting at the photographer.

Noeline has a similar pose for administering medicine. First, so as not to surprise by swooping in from the side, you make eye-level greetings, kneeling or squatting down to meet the sitting or laying resident. Establish a gaze, an endearment, for the purpose of this moment—take what you must, what is good for you—followed by a tender kiss to the cheek. It's enough to make you swallow the pill.

"I was only married six months when we went to Robben Island in 1973."

"It was fresh, fresh then!"

"Fresh, fresh! And so we started *our* journey."

~

Looking at a map, Robben Island appears much farther out in the Atlantic Ocean than ten kilometers (or six miles) northwest of Cape Town's presently glittering touristic Victoria & Alfred Waterfront. The island is surrounded by jagged reefs and long-sunken ships and has been inhabited by shifting populations of seabirds, seals, penguins, social pariahs, and prisoners since the earliest days of colonial settlement.

It is the site of the first prison to hold Indigenous peoples whom whites did not see as sovereign—the Khoi leader Autshumo and his niece, whose name remains unknown aside from Krotoa, or !Orolõas, meaning "Ward-girl," reflecting her role of interpreting between the European settlers and her people. The island has also housed "lepers," the "insane," and other medically institutionalized peoples, and, most famously, the maximum-security prison detaining oppositionists to the National Party's apartheid rule.

It also takes a village to maintain such institutions, ordinary men and women whose daily labors of dock work, deliveries, gardening, and childcare sustain the families of the people who sustain the carceral complex, the people who tear others' families apart.

Following the apartheid state's raid on their headquarters in Rivonia and subsequent treason trial, Mandela and seven other men of the ANC and Communist Party were sent to the island in 1964 to live out life sentences. Their arrival also marked the prison's expansion. Blocks D, C, B, and A were newly built—D for political prisoners—which now sound more to me like the wings of Grace.

Mandela himself wrote of those early years, "Simply, white prison staff were usually of Afrikaner stock, ill-educated and powerful. These were mainly young men and women"—women, however, who have never been previously named or discussed in this carceral tale—"the likes of whom had prompted James Baldwin's observation that 'ignorance, allied with power, is the most ferocious enemy justice can have.'"[5]

Conditions were brutal. Prisoners were tortured—beaten, starved, some sometimes nearly buried alive, their heads pissed on by guards. Many died. Throughout the 1960s, the numbers of the prison grew with new detainees from anti-apartheid and colonial struggles across Southern Africa. They organized hunger strikes and other protest actions against their conditions. Their smuggled-out letters and the very few visitors' accounts drew global attention, leading the International Committee of the Red Cross (ICRC) to send inspector Godfrey Senn to meet Mandela and others in April 1967.[6] They discussed the prisoners' living conditions and health related to prison labor—constipation and skin problems from crap diets, baton beatings, stress hernias, hypertension, permanently damaged tear glands from smashing limestone in the quarry. Prisoners successfully petitioned the administration to relieve men over the age of sixty from this specific duty.[7]

Me: "Prison ages you, Noeline," reminded again of grassroots groups in America that advocate for the release of aging people in prison—their aging accelerated and lives shortened by the institution's ordered savagery.

"Of course it does. You miss your family, you don't know anything about your finances, you don't know anything about your family. Unless it was very tragical thing, like death or birth in their family, we didn't want to tell them news that would upset them unnecessarily. They've got enough to work through."

168   GOD'S WAITING ROOM

Senn's reports helped to build international pressure for improved medical treatment of the prisoners. He returned to Robben Island in August, September, and October that same year, accompanied by medical delegate Simon Burkhard. Activist and Progressive Party Member of Parliament Helen Suzman became the first woman to visit the prisoners that year, too. Following further public outrage, Colonel Willie Willemse replaced the callous Piet Badenhorst as Head of Prison in 1971 to improve Robben Island's overall conditions, encouraged by General J. C. Steyn, the Commissioner of Prisons. And after that, the state granted international organizations regularly scheduled inspections.

Noeline and Rickus rode the waves of these changing political-carceral conditions to their new life on the island, both working for Correctional Services, around 1974. They were given a little house next to the sick bay among a small community of some five hundred married and single individuals working and living there. Rickus worked the political prisoners' finances.

"There were lots of donations coming in," Noeline explains. "The political prisoners were not poor people. They had personal tastes. Say, for instance, oh, one little example, was that they didn't want to use the toothpaste we gave them, so they ordered their own. So, he handled all that, seeing that the demands were met."[8]

(It is not too much to ask for. Given everything else.)

"And me, Casey, I was the first woman to walk in and work there since they opened it. They looked at me like, 'Are you real or are you a ghost?'"

Noeline's duties are glimpsed by Fran Lisa Buntman in an interview with Willemse who described changes in wardens' practices as paralleling that of medical staff working on the island: They "still segregated prisoners on racial lines . . . but had a very strong emphasis that prisoners have to be dealt with in . . . the spirit of the international standard which asks of staff to be professional, to regard his clients the same way as the nursing sister would be regarding patient, and not to ask what your politics are, what your religion is, what your ethnicity is, but to deal with them as human beings and apply policy."[9]

Better treatment was both a policy application and a political calculation. Mandela's former guard Christo Brand wrote, "It was better to take care of Mandela's health than have him die a martyr" in prison, as other detainees had due to extreme environmental conditions.[10]

"Was it just Correctional that employed you?"

"And the Department of Health and the Red Cross," she says, brushing away a fly that's come in through Jane B.'s window, "those two were also my direct supervisors. The most interesting thing for me was to work with the Red Cross. They were just so many steps above us"—her ringed hand passes above her reddened hair—"and they wanted their clients up there, too. TB tests, dentist and physician exams. I had an X-ray machine, so we took them every three months, and sputum tests. They wanted to see that the men were well looked after—if they got healthy food, fresh water and the like because the water was very salty. You know salt water

NOELINE 169

is not good for the body. It causes hypertension. We made sure the kitchen was hygienic, the food clean, the bedding nice. It was all kept on file. So, when they came, we had it ready for them to see. We were trying to be preventive. And if this work wasn't done—trouble!"

"Almighty. It's a lot to do"—and for multiple organizations at that, I imagine.

"Bright and early, in the mornings, early, 7 o'clock, was my starting time."

Mandela himself depicted the Robben Island hospital ward in a colored lithograph. The row of softened beds lies below rows of small windows, the walls chartreuse. Of this picture, he wrote, "On Robben Island, political and general prisoners were kept well apart. The only place where we could talk and share information with other inmates was in the prison hospital—and that thereby became more than just an infirmary. The hospital I have sketched here served as a vital link between us and the rest of the world. Through the hospital, news about our families, our friends, the struggle and everyday events outside the prison would trickle through."[11]

The news that Rickus and colleagues avoided telling them or hoped they'd forget about, rather. "These memories, like this sketch are filled with joyous colours," Mandela concluded.[12]

One writer, describing chartreuse the elixir as a verdant spring-like "sickly-green" with a taste "harsh and punishing, like medicine," also notes that "hordes" of people misremember this color for another—something blood-red-like. She says it's due to the "Mandela Effect."[13]

"In the morning, I'd go to give them their medicine," Noeline begins to list again, "check to see if anybody's sick from the night before—more people get sick at night, neh—if everybody's alright, nobody's lying in the bed with flu. I did their fissure therapy and dressings for injuries from playing football, rugby, tennis, cricket, and the like. Then, on to the medium-security prison which had the short-term prisoners. Remember, I always had a warden with me because I never carried a key."

Unlike here. I am surprised too at first to hear about sports at a prison but then recall that like the hospital ward, Mandela also depicted Robben Island's tennis courts, partly inspired by black American tennis legend Arthur Ashe.[14]

"After them, I went back to the sick bay for the members," she continues, meaning the residents of the prison's little staff village, "to do my rounds, weigh babies, inject babies, and all that. The worst I saw there was a ruptured uterus, seven months pregnant."

Jane's TV plays a rerun of the decades-long Afrikaans soap opera *7de Laan*—I guess the series is also coming to its storied end. It segues to a commercial for bargains on baby formula and chocolate bars at a green cross–branded pharmacy chain. We leave her behind. On to the also-oxygenated Mims, Johnny's girlfriend. The mask comes down for three pills to go in. After that, Eunice gets two. Eugene gets three and ointment for where his ring-finger nail should be. Trish, a lozenge and Panado.

"Did you work alone?" In Grace, she's at the top of the chain of command, or Sister Marina or Sister Janice, depending who's on duty. Then the auxiliary nurses, then the caregivers. Angel has the final say.

"There was a medical team, male medics, and me. I trained some of the political prisoners to also be medics—to work in the dispensary for me, packing the tablets, doing the filing. I had four or five of them. We had an ambulance. We were enough to, to meet the needs. The physicians and urologists and the highly specialized people like that couldn't come to the island. The District Surgeon did once a week from Cape Town in the morning to consult with us and the inmates and go back in the afternoon.[15] They were well looked after, but they had no freedom."

I remember taking a tour of Robben Island in 2004, ten years after the country's first free elections and Mandela's ascent to the presidency. The tour guides at that time were former prisoners. One of the guides told me and the group—a dozen bewildered white and black American college students—that he'd been electrocuted by a guard until he defecated. It was punishment for receiving a suspicious letter from his family, assessed by a staff member to be communicating something of political importance.

"But it was awful for them, Noeline."

"It's true too. It's not a lie. I've been there, and I saw it. It was difficult because you've got the discipline side of things and the medical side of things. And discipline does not always agree with what medicine does. So, you were in a consistent fight for standing up and saying, 'Listen, this is what I'm trained for. These are my qualifications. I will respect and abide by you when it comes to discipline, but you, do not interfere with my work. Ever."

"It was as if the wardens are just making work for you. Because the conditions were bad, their health suffered, and then you end up treating them. It's a back and forth."

"But I was cheeky. They couldn't circle up with me. I used to say to the commanding officer, 'Here's my certificate—four years of training and a degree—where's yours?' They sewed up fast!"

Toe-to-toe. Boots. Barking. At first bite, nursing is mostly women's work—Bethal's the only man on staff here. And prison is mostly men's work. Correctional nursing confounds this gendered divide that's built into the institution. Keep sexes separate both there—"there were no women wardens," she says, and there were no women prisoners—and here—unless you're a married couple like the Geldenhuyses, the Malans, others down in the cottages.

"In those days, we worked a special boat in the middle of the night. Say someone had terrible pneumonia or bronchitis, something I wasn't capable of handling. I'd tried all the antibiotics I had and other things, but now they'd need a drip. So, I'd find the crew of that boat and say, 'Mr. So-and-so is very sick. I want two guards, and I'm going with.' If the waves were too much, they sent a helicopter. And if the wind was too much, they sent an old Cessna. I was there to stabilize oxygen, band them in. I felt it was my responsibility. The guards didn't see it that way, but I knew it was what I had to do."

"Eleven years with some of these men," I reckon, "How could you not?"

"I said to myself, 'Why must this man be alone when he is sick? I don't want to be alone when I am sick.' No one wants that. So, I was there, holding their hand when they got to the hospital on the mainland. It was Somerset Hospital"—where they also sent women of the island village to have their babies—"When we got there and they saw the men holding on to me, saying, 'Don't leave me, don't leave me,' those white nurses would look at me like. . . . I'd just think to myself, 'Bugger off!'"

Do no harm.

And yet the meeting of her colleagues' eyes, I imagine, set her on fire. "It's incredible. Like Matron Pfaff at Garden City Hospital. They couldn't believe what they saw," I envision. "Do you think they were . . . 'resentful' is not the right word, but asking themselves, 'How could she help Mandela and these other men?'"

"They said to me that I'm a . . . well, I'm not allowed to say that word. They told me I was a . . ."

Turning the corner, the med cart veers to meet an end table with a vase of fake gladioli—the floor's still a bit wet from a recent mop, we guess. A metal tray holding paper towels on the cart's lower shelf spins out like a flying saucer and lands on the tiling.

The sharp percussion censors what I think she'll say and makes my skin crawl. I usually say "sorry" when things fall apart.

But something's changed in me at this point in the tour. There's nothing to be sorry for now—me or anyone else here maybe. I believe we're too far gone to worry about forgiveness. My lower back stretches uncomfortably to reach the paper towels. She restarts:

"I said to them, 'This is what I'm trained for. This is what I'm getting paid for. Do you see the inside of their hands? The soles of their feet? They are white. They didn't paint themselves black.'"

Maybe an appeal in colorism was a good counterpunch among white people back then as it is now for Angel and some of the other white people here. It still is for a lot of white people today, not caring if someone is, say, "purple, yellow, or polka-dotted"—it's just the "person" that matters in their postracial fantasy.

She turns over the little Tower of Babel pill cups that toppled in the crash, recollecting and recounting the pills.

"You know, when the prisoners were sitting and eating their meals, I used to talk to them about medicine and things, because the political prisoners were highly intelligent people. And I'd say to them in these sessions, 'Listen. I didn't put you here. I don't know why you're here. And I don't want to know.' Nelson Mandela once said to me, "Please read the Rivonia Trial.' And I said, "No, I don't want to."

"You didn't want to?"

"No," sternly. "I am here to look after you—your physical well-being. I am here to care for you. I'm not interested in the political situation. I don't carry a

172   GOD'S WAITING ROOM

gun. I don't carry a key. I only carry injections and medications. So, I don't want to know."

Self-made oblivion. Maybe for self-protection.

"The respect I got from those people, Casey, you will never understand. It was because I gave them my time. I wasn't judgmental. To me, and my husband, they were human beings. I felt that when we would sit together and watch movies, having coffee and rusks together, and those things. They would try to tell me their stories, about what was happening politically, and I said to them, 'Don't talk to me about politics, please, because I don't know what you're talking about. It is not my field, and I am not interested.' I told them, 'I was nineteen when I worked with my first African man,' and they said, 'Oh!' because they knew I meant I worked with their private parts. 'Of course,' I said, 'when you nurse, you learn to catheter.' People are in need."

"Indeed."

"This is about the human being. I used to say to them, 'Apartheid, yes, I know it. I was born in that era. I didn't ask for it. But I want to prove to you that I am not a racist.'"

I hear myself say, "Yes, I know" to her—it's not a disconfirmation of what she's saying, and yet it is. I want to know where she is going now in the tale, and where she thinks she stood with respect to these atrocities, before today.

Angel walks past us in the other direction, this time folder-less. Behind her are Precious and Yolanda, now more jovial with each other and chatting in siSwati— something about someone's husband doggedly coming home from a long trip.

Noeline's stopped re-collecting the spilled pills. She pivots. Her look meets mine, then drifts past me. It's become serious.

"The day that I left Robben Island, it was in the middle of the night. They wanted no one to know there were three political prisoners on that boat, you see. They were being transferred to Pollsmoor Prison, and we went along with them. I sent my children ahead first, and then the furniture. And one of the wardens from security phoned me and said, 'Please, don't get on the boat yet. Come to the prison. Walter wants to see you'—Walter Sisulu."

"My God."

"Walter was there. Oliver Tambo was there. A lot of them. I want to cry when I think about it."

In seconds, the soft flesh around her eyes visibly, gently swells. She's suddenly in true tears. Of course, I've now forgotten the takeaways of that oral history methods book I read, written by a theologian, with a chapter titled "What to Do When an Interviewee Cries."[16]

"Casey. He took my arms. I mean, he put his arms out to and hug my arms on each side, and said, 'We all know—God knows—what you've done for us. We'll never forget you.' They were crying. I was crying. I said to him, 'Please, get up, man, don't be standing like you are on your knees like that, you should only be on your knees to pray.'"

"'Well,' he said, 'I'm praying now to say thank you to you.'"

NOELINE

"It was traumatic. It was. If I think about it, I see that old face and white hair, the rimples in his face."

She recomposes her own with one of paper towels from the cart I've ripped away to hand her.

"Sorry. It's hard to talk about. The boat couldn't leave because of us holding them up. And when I got to the boat, there was a huge arrangement of flowers. For me."

Writing about victims of the apartheid state's violence who testified at the Truth and Reconciliation Commission, South African psychologist Pumla Gobodo-Madikizela explained that past events become inextricably tied to the present in people's storytelling. They cannot be construed as a basic reconstruction of facts—and here too, Oliver Tambo was never imprisoned on Robben Island, despite Noeline's claiming his presence that night.

After hearing hundreds of testimonies, Gobodo-Madikizela concluded that traumatic memories of the past, when retold in the present, reflect a range of impactful, often invasive experiences rather than a neutral reconstruction of historical facts. "The lived experience of traumatic memory becomes a touchstone for reality," she wrote, "and it tells us more about how people try to lead a normal life after such a trauma."[17]

Other touchstones Noeline tells me this day:

Treating shipwrecked, hypothermic Chinese fisherman with blankets and old brown brandy; treating limbs of prisoners crushed in the construction-related collapse of the old foghorn; treating a dozen-plus prisoners dead one afternoon from drinking from a drum of paraffin that had washed ashore.

These touchstones all too brightly whiten one's visions of reality—visions that include the most extraordinary others. The dead, as ghosts or ancestors, forever linked to the survivors, the living, and people who were not even there.

"Goodness!"

Med pass ends. She hands off the cart to the caregiver who's joined us.

"Rinse the cups, toss the gauze," she tells her.

Back to Bea's room now—again, the ninety-four-year-old who passed last week. It's already mostly bare. The closet has a few hangers and two robes. A box with a Bible, a hot-water pad. In the end-table drawer, a receipt from Spar for salted macadamias.

Here's a note from one Barbara Jean, a friend of Bea's daughter—it says, "Happy Easter, Luvie," and there's a phone number.

"It's hard, Noeline. There's Mom and Dad, and then there's me. I just think, what will I be able to do for them when the time comes, you know?"

"You don't have to do something when the time comes, Casey."

I know what she meant—"You do it now."

"There's nothing nicer than a phone call," she says. "Pick up the phone and say, 'Mommy, I love you.' Tell them they're important. Tell them you love them."

"They're doing some practical things," I share. "They've downsized to a smaller place, kind of like the cottages here for the folks who don't need full assistance yet. Someone else can take care of the garden, or the snow for them. But I know what you mean, it's giving love in the meantime."

"They must know and acknowledge it. They must know in their heart that while they're here, you are thinking of them. Talk to them. And if you've got the time, go to them."

"I live sort of far from them, so Thanksgiving maybe. It's like a braai for us"—I make the bad comparison—"I mean, if you did it with a huge turkey."

"We'd eat that at Christmas!"

Cleaning more, the room's barer now. The closet robes folded and slipped into a paper bag. They'll keep the Bible for the room's new occupants. The second bed will need a mattress pad and sheets. Both beds will get scrubbed down.

The end-table drawer's emptied. I fold the note from Barbara Jean and pass it to Noeline. She looks at me knowingly, scraps the woman's final message to the wastebin.

"Did doing geriatrics, palliative, prepare you for this? This place?" I ask the final question.

"Well . . . my father, he died of liver cancer. I saw him getting yellow, thinner, getting helpless, frustrated, depressed. As if he didn't feel like living anymore. I got a caregiver for him because my mother had her grandchildren to look after. She walked him, dressed him, fed him. But I saw what a caregiver actually meant to him. He was never alone."

An agency or travel nurse, maybe—someone like Bethal or Goodness, one day maybe—with just one soul to look after on this contract.

"He was only seventy-six when he died. My mom was eighty-two. Same story where her organs backed up and she needed care. I realized it was essential for them not to be alone. And that tomorrow is another end. So I sat with my father on his bed, and I said to him, 'Are you ready? Is there anything you want me to do for you?' And then he said to me, 'My circle is completed.'"

"I was lying with him on the bed. He closed his eyes, turned his head, and he was gone."

"My God," I whisper.

"Peaceful, happy, realizing what was happening with him, and telling me so. Up to this day, when I sit here with these people who are about to die, I say to them, 'Do you feel like you've achieved everything in your life that you wanted? Is your circle completed?' Some say 'yes', and some say 'no,' or, 'I want you to do this for me,' this and that. That is life," she ends.

"Life is a circle."

"And precious. It is precious—a blink and it's over. After fifty years of nursing I can still remember my first day when I walked into the ward in Oudtshoorn. I can still remember how those brown shoes squeezed my feet, and the starch uniform with this belt and things"—jangling epaulettes—"It feels like yesterday."

~

"Hello?"—I'm calling Noeline on Facebook Messenger, on her daughter Cristina's account.

"Casey, I quit. It was time."

Gugu and Yolanda stayed late at the week's end to help her do the scrub-down. Monday came. A man moved in, not black. Angel's executive decision.

Noeline knew when she saw the leather-jacketed, curly-haired daughter—the one who toured with Marina—come early for the final walk through for her father's new room-home.

"I said to her, 'You see these hands? These hands washed this room, and now you come and put a white one in here? You are a racist! You're going to jail, mama. I'll open up this whole thing and show the town what's really going on here!"

It was heated. Her son encouraged her leave. He works in HR.

She says they're still friends, though, she and Angel. It's a small town.

"What a mess, Noeline. People have problems with these things. We only just had our first black president a few years ago, and *that* was hard for some of them— to change. They're hard-asses."

"Darling, they must get over it."

The Circle

Around 5:10 P.M., Miss Frikkie began to sing. The Sisters know this song—wet, arrhythmic, and percussive, like a rattle, made by water welling in the throat as one's ability to swallow reflexively lets go. It's the sound of death's pull and a sign for staff to begin the move.

Noeline, Precious, and I hover at the bed. Their hands retract the guardrail. Free from the metal bar, the dying woman's soft world tumbles out, blankets' folds bending prayerfully. One touches my pant leg.

Noeline, wearing white today, leads confidently. Having moved through her career from prison hospital to old age home, to this final fenced-in little world, a bed with guardrails, she leans in. Again, never speak to older adults from their head's side, I learned from her—it's disorienting to them. Meet them face-to-face. Her glasses slide down just a bit to the tip of her nose as she cranes to ask:

"Sweetness, tell me, is your circle completed?"

Frikkie doesn't answer the question. Noeline leans back. Her glasses stick at the nose tip. We reassess. Precious releases a sliver of chipped ice into Frikkie's mouth. Breath pulses over the precipice of her dry lips at a slower tempo than the rattling. Noeline dips a rubber-gloved finger into a small jar of petroleum jelly next to a jar of African potato creme. Daintily, she traces Frikkie's mouth with the balm.

"It's just cosmetics, sweetness."

Because she's not speaking—or maybe just not in sounds can we hear—we start the circle ourselves. Even if Frikkie is in this room and this chapter's protagonist, us three—Noeline, Precious, and me—have to narrate a script of her life instead. She moves in and out of what the sociologist Erving Goffman called the "participant framework," meaning as we talk with this nonspeaking woman, we shift between speaking in second- to third-person—"you" to "her."[1] We subtly recalibrate to make sure we are talking *with* her somehow rather than *about* her—language is funny like this.

THE CIRCLE

I find I do this when talking to someone about someone they've loved who's passed, saying things like, "Oh, she misses you." Like Precious told Andrew before: "Dickie is always watching."

What we narrate about Frikkie lacks the immediate corroboration her family might offer if they were there with us in the room. They are off in other cities and the United States like Bethal surmised. Still, we feel this script is needed—an elaboration, a celebration, or a re-envisioning of her life history. We, and the atmosphere of the room, behold her remaining. In story form, we perform her life as a deathbed confession.

To tell the story, we use the words that Frikkie once told me about her life.

Or maybe it was another woman's words, I now wonder—at another time, on another day here maybe. I can't remember.

But I hear it now. Parts of a past conversation that struck me, were written down, lingering still. Now floating back into mind, the time and place of this room. The nurses, do they hear her words too?

Do you?

(*"What about my life, Casey?" she says to me. "I can't remember much anymore. But everything is alright with me. I'm easygoing. If it's alright with me it's alright with you. There's nobody coming in here making a mess of us, no one bilking us. Life's been all right."*)

The circle is a universal symbol. In its lineation, it forms an unending thing. To counter its infinitude, we demarcate a point as its beginning and end—a start and finish. Circles convey containment, completion, wholeness. In black communities here, circles reckon enclosure as they form the shape of houses and homesteads in their architecture. They order mind, heart, and family. The circle is a symbol for these communities in relations of chieftaincy.

"*Bamba*" (Hold this), says Precious to me.

She hands me a few melting ice chips in a white emesis basin.

"Frikkie is pray-er, she is. She was like an angel when she prayed with our Sisters. That's why her name is Engela," Noeline says to us, recalling what's on the dying woman's birth certificate. Frikkie's a nickname.

Like the nurses' gold necklaces, Frikkie also has a cross. It's wooden and suspended on the wall above her bed. If we extend its arms and post, extend it beyond Jesus's death-by-crucifixion, the lines of the cross come to structure a diameter of sorts—the spokes of her circle turning as a wagon wheel.

Frikkie's ancestors drove their covered wagons through this area looking for founts or springs for their farms and animals—the Afrikaans words for these waters (*fontein, spruit*) adjoin the names of towns they built among and fortified against the people who were here first—Nelspruit renamed Mbombela, Klipfontein renamed eNgwenyameni, two Tweefonteins renamed Somaroboro and Phumula, respectively—ghosts of each place's founders commingling still.

The new names don't connote water like the old ones did, but Precious's ancestors knew these places and pools are vital. Spirits live in their rivers, alight from the sky in the rain, stir the healing waters the settlers likened in song to the biblical Bethesda.[2] They cleanse for some trespass,

For a rebirth.

(*"My mother would ask us, 'Are you clean enough? Are you happy? Would you like to go here or there with us?'—errands and holidays. She was always raising us up and wanting to know if we were happy. That was important to her, that her children were happy. We were happy. I think we were. She was just a housewife. That is what I want you to know. . . . And my father, he was a very happy man. But you know men, he hardly had anything to do with us. He spoke to my mom, and she decided then what to do with us. But it was very nice to have a dad. I couldn't imagine not having one until after he died. But we were very happy family."*)

Frikkie was born in a house made of field stones, in 1932. Henrik van den Berg, her father, and her mother, Marie, were pious people, members of the Dutch Reformed Church. The sect took off in small settler towns like theirs of Machadodorp, now Ntokozweni, originally named for a Portuguese colonial major and railroad engineer. Henrik worked for the railroad that connected their town to what is today Mozambique. In 1900 the town was temporarily made the capital for the Afrikaner nation-state during the Second Anglo-Boer War (1899–1902). Marie and Henrik's parents had survived, and the new Union of South Africa was founded in its wake in 1910. Their family's thriving in that place and time felt preordained.

"She's her husband's girl," Precious smiles.

(*"As a girl, there was nothing that I hated in school. Not a boarding school, but I can't remember. . . . Then I had my first boyfriend. . . . But I can't remember if I was still in school, sixteen or seventeen. But I enjoyed it very much. I loved it. Everything I did I loved. My mom says, 'Engela, you mustn't love him too much because you must first take your exams.' I said, 'Mom, you don't need to worry.'"*)

One of Frikkie's long fingers is laden with a ring, a princess-cut diamond. She excels, or excelled, in knitting. Her mother taught her. She showcased winterwears made from lambswool at the Easter fair.

In 1948, a blond twenty-two-year-old World War II veteran, Frederik Thuynsma, took the train to visit his aunt in Machadodorp. At the fair he bought a dyed-yellow scarf from sixteen-year-old Engela. They married a year later in the van den Berg's church and bought a plot for a small farm on land reallocated for white settlement by the national government. "Frikkie" is a nickname for Frederik, and he went by "Rik." "Frikkie" is what his aunt and her parents called her as she went about her new bridal life. On Saturdays she rode a carriage to the little railroad town, gardened the churchyard. On Sundays she grilled trout wrapped in bay leaves.

THE CIRCLE   179

"Melina said she made the best cherry liqueur for Christmas," adds Precious to her story.

Marina told me that Frikkie once told her about making the liqueur, that Frikkie's daughter Melina loved it. Again, alcohol's a no-no at Grace, even on holidays and family visits. The drink languishes on my mind's tongue though. I'd read about it, too, in Zakes Mda's novel *The Madonna of Excelsior*, about miscegenation in another South African small town like Frikkie's and the children that came from "inter-racial" relations.[3] The Immorality Act that criminalized this love passed in 1950, making a crime of those born of it. Marina also told me Frikkie raised the children to ride horses. And pigs.

Yellowing pictures of Frikkie's children, Melina, Dirk, and Frederick Jr., line the wall next to the hanging cross.

Noeline, to the dying woman: "We know your children love you. We are family here too. Every one of us is God's child."

(*"I had three children, two boys and a girl, and they went to the best schools. They were very happy. The boys played tennis and she was in swimming. They all went to university, and they did good and finished their degrees. I said to them, 'Don't mind at all where you land or where you're going. As long as you learn and know something about something, I don't mind if you leave me.' So, they left."*)

The railroad via Machadodorp ends where white sands wash into the Indian Ocean. It begins in Pretoria. Frikkie's children rode there for their studies to attend the main university campus ornamented with coats of arms of woodland stags. It expanded threefold in the 1960s as national education policies enriched schools for whites and delimited the curriculum for citizens of color. Her daughter now lives "overseas," a professor of hydrogeology at UPenn or Penn State in the United States, a field that's been lucrative in South Africa for generations given its usefulness to the mining industry. One son works in insurance, the other in HR. Bruce says their debit orders always come in on time to cover Mom's stay.

(*"My dad's sister played such beautiful piano. I learned to play from her. Or maybe I learned it myself."*)

"She's a great piano player. We'll send the kids the video," I say. I had watched a video on Bruce's phone of Frikkie playing the piano—she would have at the worship service today instead of Barra, had she been up to it, they told me. The video showed the whole sitting room listening attentively as Frikkie tickled the ivories—no oontz-oontz. It was a long time ago.

"We're like her family here. It doesn't matter who you are. We are her family too," says Precious.

Frederik, "Rik," passed away three years ago. After his wartime military stint, he worked for the police in some form.

When some of the women residents get aggressive here, the caregivers joke that they learned it from their late husbands—like Rik, perhaps—men who *may* have done unspeakable things in the past. Gugu and others told me, on the side, that Frikkie was sometimes the most aggressive in her last few months—angry, lashing out. Her antics went beyond "performing."

"She must've been a lady-baas . . . Vlakplaas," one of the staff joked.

No one laughed at that one.

It is a word that means "shallow farm." It is a real place and sits on an unassuming dusty parcel about twenty kilometers from the University of Pretoria campus, ringed by a few grey hillocks.

It's not a good word to say here or anywhere in South Africa. It's like opening a grave. Maybe like the bare patch where the ancestors lie outside in Grace's yard. Saying it, or talking about it, will resurface a difficult story. And more.

(*"You know, the black and white people don't mind being together at all as they were years and years ago,"* she says, *"You know blacks would never associate with us and us with blacks. You know what it was like."*)

And before we learn "what it was like," one last trigger warning:

This shallow farm was occupied by a small group of white men—high-school-educated police officers, none of whom the staff can be sure were Frikkie's or the other tannies' late husbands—and a few black men who were "converted" to join their cause of sussing out anti-apartheid activists and operatives. They were underground.

The white men of Vlakplaas bombed offices and homes. They slaughtered a family of five in Botswana, and a group of eight in Lesotho, including a husband and his unarmed wife, whose one-year-old daughter was left alive and alone next to her dead mother. They blew up the car of their own black colleague, whom they suspected of double-crossing them. They sent a young lawyer a bomb hidden in a cassette player, which took off his head while he sat at home with his wife. They kidnapped an apolitical security guard, tortured him for information on his guerrilla brother, and, realizing he knew nothing, bashed in his head with a shovel and hid the body.[4]

"*Ungiphe*" (Gimme that). Precious takes back the washcloth and vomit basin.

A man named Eugene de Kock ran the farm for most of the 1980s. He was one of two such killers employed by the apartheid government who was denied amnesty at the Truth and Reconciliation Commission, a seven-year public forum held after apartheid ended to air these atrocities. De Kock was then imprisoned. He was the main interview subject of Pumla Gobodo-Madikizela's tome *A Human Being Died That Night* about the impossibilities of forgiving such crimes, de Kock's motivations, and whether he or not he was truly apologetic. Comparing him to the doctors who conducted experiments on prisoners in the Holocaust, she assessed that he was.[5]

After his interviews with Gobodo-Madikizela, de Kock met some of his victims' families. One was Marcia Khoza, the daughter of Portia Shabangu, an activist in

THE CIRCLE 181

the South African National Student Congress. In 1989, Portia, Thabo Mohale, and Derek Mashobane traveled near here to then-Swaziland thinking they were headed for underground resistance training with the ANC. There, in the woods near Bhunya, they were ambushed.[6] Portia was shot multiple times with a semi-automatic rifle. "De Kock checked her pulse by placing his pinky finger on her eyelid, and then shot her twice in the head again."[7]

The day they met at his prison, de Kock and Khoza shook hands. She gave him a book with a note inside:

"I have been hurt and had a rough childhood without my mother, since 12 Feb 1989. I am healed and free from bitterness and hatred. I freely and fully forgive you, and I am ready to help others to heal. Let the power of peace and forgiveness guide you, be with you and others for the rest of our lives. You're totally forgiven."

According to Khoza, de Kock cried.[8]

(*"You see another person with another color, and you know he's not your type. I think that's what I thought," Frikkie reasons. "Now I don't mind going on with him, because now we don't mind at all. Where blacks are, the white people are, and where the white people are the black people are. We don't mind at all."*)

"I know you don't want it, sweetness. No more water. No more now," Noeline whispers to Frikkie.

After apartheid, Louis Smit, a born-again Christian and white supremacist and his wife Luisa were appointed by the Department of Public Works as the shallow farm's caretakers. In 1996, the Smits permitted one hundred sangomas from the Indigenous Knowledge Secretariat to do libations and appease the ancestors of the murdered, both there and beyond.[9] The Smits refused to leave when the government then tried to turn the farm into a museum and a place to grow plants used in these healers' medicine. The couple transferred the property instead to their friends who opened a drug rehabilitation center. That eventually closed, and the shallow farm was turned over to the Ministry of Arts and Culture.[10]

Whites still own Grace, the surface of the plot of earth we stand on now, and many of the plots around us—the macadamia and citrus farms, the forest estates.

What lies beneath the surface can never be owned. At least not in ways they would understand.

Frikkie moved to Grace when Rik passed, when she was left alone on her bridal farm plot with a few contracted laborers. According to Noeline, Frikkie's children reasoned that it was too dangerous for her to age-in-place there.

Earlier today, Johnny's roommate Johann told me a story that showed me this reasoning pervades the white community around here. One evening, he was braaiing with his son and daughter-in-law when five masked men drove up in pickup trucks and attacked them. They pushed Johann and his son to the ground, beating the son and daughter-in-law with a rifle buttstock. With a finger on a trigger, for what Johann recollected was two hours, one demanded that he turn over his guns—375s, big rifles. Three of the five were police officers, Johann said, their identities revealed when they were killed while raiding another farm.

"You can die quickly" when looking too deeply into such business, like Goodness said.

Johann moved to Grace after that. For Frikkie, too, and other older people across the racial spectrum—in their children's eyes at least—aging-in-place, or alone at least, can be a security issue.

(*"Now, we don't mind each other in here because we are equals. We're all the same, black and white."*)

(*Me to her: "I hope it can be so."*)

(*"Unless you swear," she stammers—a choke, a hiccup. "I sometimes hear it. I worry. I say to them, why are you swearing at me? You don't get anything for doing it.' I can't give you what you want!"*)

(*"Who is swearing, tannie? One of the residents?" I think I hear Precious asking.*)

(*"I don't know. I don't know why, but I think I hear it. They're swearing. Outside here, there, they are fighting. They want ... no"—she breathes steadily now—"If they don't swear at me, I don't mind. But I don't like it. I don't like it very much at all."*)

(*"What do they say, tannie? What are they fighting about?"*)

(*"I don't know. But you must know this: I am ready to accept anything."*)

~

"17:40."

Noeline announces the time we stop giving her water; a futility since she began her song. Precious writes it down with a red pen. Nurses use twenty-four-hour or military time.

"Let me call Melina—or leave a message. It's what time in the States?" she asks me. 11:40—a six-hour difference.

Beneath the cross, Frikkie emits a dispassionate gaze, lids barely unclosing, her eyes crescents the color of dried cornflower. Glaucoma pervades. Noeline once told me that a dying person's eyes can also look cloudy like a fish's.

Dinner's already been plated. Today, it's brown bread with butter, a tomato slice, a frankfurter. Like yesterday, nothing's left on her bedside table.

Shift will end at 6:00 P.M. The next shift is here, Janice again and two aides. They all changeover with the evening security detail—a lone guard.

Someone else will watch her.

Someone will listen to the song, or hear its end.

Someone will wait.

Confessions

"You're still here?"

"You are too."

The staff have already left. We've said our goodbyes. They're on the 6:00 A.M.–6:00 P.M. shift, yes, but the stories of roadblock protests on the way back to the townships swayed Noeline—heartsore. She let them go early. "How would you like it if you didn't get home till past 8 and the kids are still waiting for food?" she asked rhetorically. "Men!"

(I'm asleep by the time Charlie's home from the 4:00 P.M.–4:00 A.M. shift at the hospital.)

To the residents, too, we've said our goodbyes—Andrew, Yvonne, Mama Zulu, the Janes, Frikkie, the rest.

Down A wing, B wing, C, most of their rooms are shut. Under a few, a soft line of light marks the threshold between door and floor.

Some are likely still wake inside, some asleep with the lights on. Some face the home's western perimeter, those who each day watch the sun set.

A soft rush meets my face, a breeze from an ajar door, or someone's exhale, whispering *"Lishona 'langa, ulibambe lingashon'"* (Don't let the sun go down on you)—an African saying, siSwati, not Elton John's—meaning "Save yourself from retribution." I turn.

Angel—she's sighed that "it's-been-a-long-day" sigh.

"Same," I breathe out, "I'm ready to take this mask off."

We've all let them slide down a little during the tour. Still, let's keep them on for good measure.

"It's a must, yes," she agrees, "but we all let down our defenses. You'll be safe enough. Trust me," she winks, "and maybe, when you're back, we won't need to wear these damn things!"

"I hope so," I say, truthfully, "and I will be"—these kind of road trips and their projects take a while, sometimes seven years or so.

Angel smiles suggestively, "You could stay awhile longer. Someone in the kitchen will fix you a plate."

I mean, I wouldn't mind a to-go box, another umphako, but doesn't she want to get out of here? It's past early dinner time. Her dogs have to be fed. But none of the jumble she had on this morning—the key lanyard, thermos, fleece—are with her now. The endorphin-high urgency that carried her into the office this morning is gone. Now, she's serene.

In this new aura, her gold cross necklace somehow shines more sharply. It's transfixing, pulling my focus from thoughts of leaving to another state of mind.

Laughing a bit to make my "No, thank you" more obvious, but keeping it sincere, I say, "I learned so much"—the stories told, the passing hours that melted into something like timelessness, the "presents"—"Everyone's been so gracious. I will never be the same."

"Grace. It's part of our name, neh? We wouldn't be like a family without it. And you have so much to write about now," she quips, eyeing my notes. "I know it will be the book that shows we are the best old age home in the country!"

I wonder if I could actually write that book. It'd be a bold review. I still haven't checked their Facebook page to see how others have rated it. I should've looked when we were stuck in the waiting room.

Still, I *could* say that it is the best place I've found thus far to learn some important lessons that can impact all of us: on how to reckon with racism at life's end, and do it through grace.

(There's a lot to say about grace according to the theologians and the like, but let's go more so with what we learned from the extraordinary people we met today.)

The souls in this out-of-the-way place are not so unlike anyone else in the modern world marred by violence and inequalities. They show us that despite a fraught past and radical differences that would pit them against each other—due of course to racism, ageism, sexism, economic inequalities, and the ways these all intersect—they still try to coexist. And they show us that despite these oppressive or difficult circumstances, they still try to give something to each other:

Grace. Here, to me, it looked like this: You're minding your business, and someone unlikeable appears before you—they walk up to you, text or call, or post something online, whatever. And in a flash, you think you know their story:

They're broken, vulnerable, struggling with some foible or problem that's personal or structural. They're poor or sick, or they're too well-off, an arrogant ass and don't know it, oblivious, or only partially aware of what's going on in the world or how they act. Maybe you knew all that beforehand about them, or it was only apparent at first sight. And now here they are, in your face—face-to-face, on your screen or on the page. What is it that you give to them in this moment and after?

CONFESSIONS

Acceptance—meaning you might tolerate them at first, for a little while at least, or in a fuller sense accept that they are like you in some shape or form despite being unlikeable. For the staff here especially, perhaps seeing that even the most irritating residents are somehow like them—that they, too, may grow older, forget, or recollect differently, dis-identify with who they once were, or begin to physically dis-integrate. Acceptance through empathy is not automatic—it's not guaranteed that someone will put themselves in your slippers or whatnot. It's just one possible outcome of a time and place and relationships with others, an outcome we've seen here at Grace. We are, by nature, social and have the innate capacity to give and receive, from affirming and empathetic ways to the grossly negative—some call this our intersubjective potential.[1]

Accepting others may be tough, of course, and even feel impossible or like doing so will kill you—maybe because this other person is so annoyingly or egregiously wrong in their actions or perspective. Or you believe they will turn on you later.

Where then will the power to accept someone so horrible come from?

One way is by what's generally called "divine grace." For some contemporary religious or spiritual types, like most people in here, the power to dole out acceptance comes as a sudden influx of some mysterious or metaphysical force. The power is said to be a gift, the force being God, the gods, ancestors, or other beings enveloped in the shadows nearby, and there's something immense and otherworldly to it. They say that by experiencing this power, you too may feel accepted, loved, or transformed.

Black liberation theologians have long meditated on the impossibilities and forms of divine grace experienced by black communities living in white-dominated societies that have not or will never accept them nor see them as fully human.[2] The Reverend Dr. Roland Hill, for example, characterizes the power of "Black Grace" as something like an Alka-Seltzer, the sodium bicarbonate and citric acid medicine for sour stomach and indigestion. Noeline doles it out here daily. Hill writes:

"When God's grace is dropped undeserved and unearned into the life [of Black people], a divine salvific reaction occurs. For Black people, grace fizzes up to replace our stolen identity"—no thanks to white supremacy—"with our new identity in Christ. The new identity is existential and experiential. It's life. This grace identity defies the reason and logic of institutionalized racism and white-washed Christianity, and Jim-Crowism because it is deemed impossible. Fizzing up from the souls of Black flocks is the grateful response," divined by God, to the sickening conditions they face.[3]

Black Grace is a sort of preventive force, Hill continues, "a restraining power holding back vengeance against a relentless oppressive society." But as it comes to dwell and work its power inside of us, metaphysically like a spirit or medically like an Alka-Seltzer, we see that it could affect any body who's been marginalized: "the essence of Black Grace is not color, but character. Character shaped on the anvil of oppression, in the fires of affliction, and the furnace of bigotry."[4]

But what if you don't believe in a divine source as kindling your power to accept others? What if you don't suffer from this kind of spiritual acid reflux?

Another way would be by what's called "secular grace."[5] In this version, the power to dole out acceptance still feels immense or extraordinary. But it actually emerges from within ourselves and our communities, rather than from the gods somewhere in the sky or encroaching dusk. It emerges because of the real-life ethical situations we find ourselves in, where you and another person, however bad or imperfect, are somehow bound together by your circumstances. It might be a situation like relationship-under-contract, perhaps—you work together, or you owe your ex-spouse alimony. Or you're both stuck in a confined place—an old age home, a prison. Or you both face a major threshold—like the end of life.

I believe it is in these shared, difficult situations that the power of acceptance emerges. It comes from recognizing that like you, anyone may become stuck, overwhelmed, vulnerable—the likelihood varies, of course—and maybe pitifully so. And at the same time, it comes from recognizing that the minds and bodies we have to move through such situations will eventually break down, by the gods' plans or the unnatural dynamics whereby our lives otherwise come to a mortal end. In the daily life of this home, these difficult situations appear in different, intertwined forms: being underpaid, facing casual-to-overtly racist comments, experiencing depression and isolation—all sadly ordinary manifestations of modern health care.

Grace as an acceptance of these difficult situations also appears in different, intertwined forms: a resignation, a shrug, a "whatever, just let them be" or "pay them no mind" sensibility. Just do your job, say "gooie more" and "goodnight," do as you're told, wipe their ass, serve the tea, politely receive it. Move on.

And yet, it is hard for the staff and residents to feel so fully detached or desensitized, despite their training or historical priming to be resigned to such situations. Some people here are genuinely close with each other in ways we could not have imagined—like a family, maybe, or friendship—despite the odds. It's mostly a gray or shadowy area between these two polar ends of total resignation and hearty friendship, an area we might call ambivalence.

Because you may be left wondering now, "Well, what's in it for me?" to be gracious to someone who's been primed to disregard you, to someone who's not in it because they actually care about you, are just going through the motions for the paycheck?

Shouldn't we *get* something when we *give* our acceptance?

Well, could it be the power of knowing you're morally superior?

No. We're not into ranking people anymore. By morals, race, gender, class, or the like.

Could it be the power of a confession? Beholding someone who comes to you in penitent admission to say "sorry," "I was mistaken," or "I'm the problem. It's me"?

No. Some anti-racists tend to find confessions like this to be mostly worthless. Confessions of white privilege—stating out loud, that you've been privileged within

CONFESSIONS

racist systems we altogether inhabit—does not do anything except to make the confessor feel better.[6] Confess, if you feel like it, just not to us, some anti-racists would say. Apologize, sure, but do something too.[7] Vote, protest, join community-based movements for abolition and empowerment. Learn and practice healing justice. Help others learn to do so. We must.

Could it be the power of forgiveness?

Maybe. Many people around the world believe forgiveness as an ethical fix of sorts is truly important.[8] But a good counterpoint from South Africa is offered by the writer Sisonke Msimang. At the first Nelson Mandela Lecture held in Amsterdam in 2019—the origin place of some of those settler-colonists we've met—Msimang argued that once apartheid ended, many white people's hearts and minds were scooped into a "cult of forgiveness" which has warped their understanding of history and the potential for what comes next.

Forgiveness should be the "humble servant of the king and queen, peace and justice," writes Msimang, rather than the driving force of politics and policies I mentioned like Obamacare, NHI, or any others that aim to change our unequal social welfare or health care systems. Talk about forgiving white people for their complicities or inactions in the face of anti-black violence assuages white people's anxieties about where they belong in a changing world. White people's comparative material advantage to people of color is not actually threatened in this changing world, and their focus on forgiveness "supersedes black people's pain" and need for justice in a reparative or restorative sense, according to Msimang. "White people in all contexts where historical wrongs have been carried out must learn that black people's lives do not center around their feelings," she says. White people "will not die if they do not receive the love from black people that they think they deserve."[9]

White people *do* die in any case and in places like Grace more so than elsewhere. Plus, the black staff members of this place also likely gave up waiting for a heartfelt or heartsore apology a long time ago—you heard so yourself. But reading between Msimang's lines, I believe the staff *do* give the residents love—just not in a way that's expected.

Sounding somewhat like the grace we've witnessed here, black liberation theologian Marvin E. Wickware Jr. writes that love can be a form of acceptance too, "acceptance of one's radical, even fundamental need for the beloved."[10] This means black and white people, all people, are part of God's beloved humanity—that is, if we believe in Him or Her, or we believe God is actually *Us* in some disaggregated form. No one is unneeded, according to Wickware Jr., even if white supremacy primes us to be believe some people are unneeded enemies whom we can do without. This priming must be acknowledged and deconstructed, and the justifiable rage that black people experience in dealing with this must be honored. White people will have to deal with the discomfort they'll feel when facing this rage. (No tears, please.)

Despite the awful, inherited past that lingers in the present in this place, a grace-like black love for white people is indeed possible, writes Wickware Jr. But it doesn't mean accepting abuse from white people or endlessly encouraging them to change. It may seem to be impossible, and, after a while, acceptance may appear as that now-familiar resignation, shrug, or "pay them no mind" attitude that many staff members showed to Grace's more problematic residents. Importantly, he concludes, love "need not demand a neat resolution or happy ending." If we are truly part of this God's universe, then white people, like all people, have capacities for moral action—capacities to give and receive, to make good on the past—and perhaps in *the* final judgment we're all waiting for, they "can truly be redeemed."[11]

More broadly then, we can see how giving grace as acceptance to sometimes-repugnant others—old racists, or whites in general, speaking as one myself—is indeed possible, without necessarily forgiving them or being "nice" per se, even if we saw that people here tend to do so.

And yet we're still left asking: what do we *get* out of all of this?

While sitting in the waiting room before, I wondered whether we might behold a new era of black empowerment in the wake of an older generation's passing, and whether their deaths mean an end to systems of white supremacy that they were complicit with or perpetuated. By now, I believe the answer is "no."

The descendants of avowed white supremacists and those who unwittingly absorb its principles will likely reproduce these systems today and tomorrow. A new era of black empowerment requires the death of such systems and ideologies—not individual people—the death or cessation of extractive practices we've inherited that undo our world socially, economically, environmentally. We need a guiding vision, of more sustainable, equitable, more-than-humanizing systems or modes of redistribution—a flourishing—that supports the most vulnerable among us and regenerates our world or creates a new one.

It will take time, and not all of us will make it that long to see it come to fruition. In the meantime, white people especially must encourage each other, rather than people of color, to interrogate their daily and long-term choices to reveal how their current position is one they've inherited—sometimes through violence—or uncritically adopted. It will take solidarity among working- and middle-class people especially, the majority of us in our modern world, to change what we have now—to mobilize our disproportionate political power to change prevailing systems that reproduce the violence of white supremacy.[12]

It will take time, and the older white people of Grace are almost out of it.

It does not mean they cannot try, but it may be too exhausting for most of them—in terms of both self-work and the structural work that politics demands. No one's offered reparations here, and most of the residents did not reflect on their role in racist oppression. Some deferred blame to their peers instead. We also heard most of the staff tell us that racist-acting residents here can't quite change their disposition, even if they wanted to. Actively making those critical, conscious changes in the world may be impossible for some due to their physical dis-integration or pains that accompany aging, as well as the psychological dis-

CONFESSIONS

identification in dementia or dreamlike states some increasingly inhabit. For some, it may be too late.

So, in the end, we see that the burden of racial reckoning at life's end is both enormous and intimate. Our abilities to reckon may be conditioned by aspects of aging. And the burden to give grace in its love-like forms of acceptance falls mainly on the shoulders of marginalized peoples within our social welfare and health care systems—the smocks, hands, and hearts of the black staff members of Grace. We see that this reckoning is racially unequal, as these systems still are the world over.

Looking at the wall clock's hands, still arrowing to 6:00 somehow, I wonder: maybe there's another way to reckon with racism at this point—by flipping the script we have about life's end and aging, and the roles we're expected to play with the script. Maybe by reckoning with ageism as it informs this script and intersects with racism, sexism, and other -isms, we can move forward—by accepting, then engaging with those aspects of aging I've called dis-integration and dis-identification.

Choosing to dye one's graying hair or to use Spanx, Botox, or anti-wrinkle cream arguably creates a different image of oneself by trying to obscure aspects of our own physical aging or dis-integration. They're actions that enable you to dis-identify as aged or make others identify or perceive you as less aged. The American anthropologist Sarah Lamb argues these actions reflect particularly Western cultural beliefs that we must age "successfully."[13] We must try hard to be fit, healthy, and beautiful so to be seen as young-despite-being-older, but we must not try "too hard" or we will be scorned for not aging "gracefully." Fewer try to age honorably or naturally or know how to accept the fallout should aging successfully not work.

Sometimes dis-identification is a passive or indirect process or more piecemeal. Due to ageism and life course changes, some older adults may need to let go of aspects of their identities that they've held dear or believed to be integral parts of themselves. In late life, for example, people might no longer be able to perform the duties of the doting mother or father, madam of the household, or boss of the workplace—identities they may have passionately owned, or stereotypes through which others saw them. Aging and frailty can also disrupt or change one's gender or racial identities or position of privilege.[14] As we age, we begin to have much less control over anything—from our bowels to when we need to go to bed. At Grace, the staff certainly don't let residents get away with *too* much or let them do much of anything on their own.

Sometimes dis-identification is an active or political process, or it has the potential to be. Acknowledging that we are differently caught within these multiple, unequal systems that shape parts of our identity, we can actively or directly let go of our investments in some of those parts. Allowing or empowering ourselves to become someone new—an un-becoming from who we believed ourselves to be or were made to be. Even in late life, we can rework aspects of our identity, by which power—gendered, racial, or political—is held or maintained,[15] even using stereotypes others hold about us to our advantage.

Not weaponizing aspects of our identity against others who are also oppressed, of course—as older white Karens are said to do against people of color—but activating those aspects as part of collaborative efforts toward material transformations that can better the lives of everyone.

Again, Sisonke Msimang helps us to see this from South Africa. In the early 1990s, Nelson Mandela was residing in Pollsmoor Prison. By then, Noeline had left Pollsmoor to go to Garden City Hospital. Mandela was effectively cut off from his ANC comrades who were still banned then in South Africa and who would have helped to shape his negotiations with F. W. de Klerk and the National Party about the transition to democracy. Neither side—ANC nor National Party—was ready.

Alone in the cell, Mandela realized he could use his institutionalized position in prison, his solitude in isolation, and others' ideas about his age, as a pretense to act: "My solitude gave me a certain liberty and I decided to do something I had been pondering for a long while: begin discussions with the government. My solitude would give me an opportunity to take the first steps in that direction without the kind of scrutiny that might destroy such efforts," that being the scrutiny and eager buzzing of his comrades who were supposed to give him the authority to begin those discussions with de Klerk about ending apartheid.[16]

He wrote further, "My isolation furnished my organization with an excuse in case matters went awry: the old man was alone and completely cut off and his actions were taken by him as individual," his ANC comrades could argue. Mandela used that isolation and the image of an institutionalized and thus incapacitated older adult to safeguard a path to black liberation. This was "the beginning of the end of the Apartheid regime," Msimang concluded. "I am here today—we are all here today—because of that splendid isolation."[17]

We will likely find ourselves in difficult situations like his one day—not prison, per se, but an insecure or temporary home, a stifled job or relationship, a waiting room of sorts. They can all feel exceptionally isolating, yes, and may be antithetical to our flourishing. But if we can't make our way out of a situation just yet, we can try to make the most of it by drawing on what we have left—time, our mortality, others' ideas about us, however stereotypical—or those mysterious forces that tend to appear around us when we face what we believe to be the end.

Indeed, if not by way of a dis-identification from who we believe ourselves to be, then the physical aspects of aging in dis-integration may be another resource for change. Returning to the question of what we get for giving grace, residents like Andrew or Mama Zulu *do* impart something important: acceptance, again, and empathy, for ourselves.

On a daily basis the residents offer their own frailty and vulnerability as embodied truths that we may all be like them one day. Maybe not that we will end up in a place like Grace nor to such a chronological age, but that they are nonetheless "us," in a basic mortal sense. Frail older adults reveal the truth that we are forever changing in interwoven physical, psychological, and spiritual dimensions, concentrated in the form of a de-muscling, thinning, or swelling body of bones, blood, and skin—maybe later, with pacemakers and stents—and that we may

CONFESSIONS

carry with us aspects of ourselves and past actions that we can't fully dispossess if we wanted to.

More critically, in each resident's passing—Bea, members of a past generation, one by one—they offer the renewed possibility for all of us to reflect on and reconsider the future of our world, and how and whether to change things or accept them as they are.

Maybe Grace's black staff members, like many others like them in our health care systems, do not need older, dying white people to remind them of their own mortality, vulnerability, and the like. They see much of it in their own communities because of what white people of all ages and white supremacy as a system itself have done to them, both past and present. Still, you can choose to disregard this counterpoint altogether if you believe it sounds like I'm making one side matter more than the other.

Maybe what we *do* get as witnesses to this case of racial reckoning at life's end is a practical demonstration of grace in action and the mysterious power it has to both hold our shared lives together and move them along. In this out-of-the-way place, we witness the practice of loving one's enemy in the sense we talked about before—tough love, without a happy ending we might expect or wish for. Love itself is rarely uncomplicated, even between married couples, parents and children, friends, and others who claim to be like-a-family. Tensions and past experiences, ranging from the traumatic to the mundane, always color or haunt our present interactions.

Grace's staff especially do the very hard, often-characterized-as-Christian-like thing of being kind to the residents who inevitably represent generations of oppression and those among them who may be overtly confrontational. Maybe I, as a white person, could have been more confrontational with those residents or others I met who spouted nasty, racist remarks—it is white people's job to do this, yes. But perhaps if I did, this tour would not have taken place.

It is remarkable, and unsettling to behold, yes. This inequality should not exist, and yet it does—for now. The theologian M. Wolff suggests we could at least give these people kudos—the ancient Greek term for glory or renown achieved through strength—for finding the power, either within themselves or from a divine source, to give grace.[18]

And as I first suggested, it might be good to give a dash of grace to older racists—maybe your own father or mother who's been whitewashed or Fox Newsified, or yearns for the good old days—just at first, as a conversation starter, to encourage them to change their tune. A warm-up to soften their rigid ideas about others before they die at least, so they might not haunt us further once they do leave this world.

In a way, we might encourage them, or anyone really, to let go of hatefulness and take on that transcendent, cosmic perspective that several residents here adopted—on what comes next, saying tomorrow is a "mystery" rather than the next day on the calendar. Most were waiting instead for the presence and judgment by a divine force they believe has existed prior to the creation of modern racial or gendered identities we've worried about. In their remaining time, they cultivate acceptance of that fate that they believe we all share. It's not a cop-out per se—that they simply shrug and do nothing *more*. It is just one way to accept their sometimes difficult situation of what the physician Atul Gawande calls "being mortal."

How they express this acceptance was not always clear. As you heard, some residents' insights on life's end were clipped, sounded garbled, or were even silent. Some sounded like a prophesy, sharing insights from their closer proximity to another world yet unseen by those of us who are further from death. Maybe what this place has shown us is that for grace to work in the wake of violence, it may require an out-of-body-and-mind state of being, a dreamlike state of catatonia or dementia where something like grace or love among enemies can emerge, where imperfect words and physical utterances are summoned as we approach and speak across the gulf that is the interpretive threshold of language itself—a deathbed confession in anticipation of what comes next.

Maybe it will be Hell, or maybe Heaven if we've accepted God and made good of ourselves as many residents suggested. For staff members, Heaven was indeed a possibility, but so was ending up in another spiritual place called "home." But, I now remember, if we die by some other way than our ancestors' or God's plan, we won't actually make it home—we'll be "spooked," as Miss Motsa said, left wandering or unmoored.

I guess once we die, we end up in different places. Instead of a multiverse, the afterlife will still be segregated as this life was.

Shit.

~

Angel butts in, "That's the point."

"Is it?"

"If you didn't figure out that I have the key to the place *you're* going after this, I don't know where you think you've been this whole time."

"But aren't we all made in His image?" I stammer. Bethal, Andrew, others said so. "How could we not all end up in same place after this?" thinking that God or whoever is waiting for us on the other side was going to be more inclusive.

"We are all made like that, sure, but let's be real, doctor."

Something like a hiccup escapes my throat.

I realize that the woman I thought I knew to be Angel—Pat's wife, Wayne's new girlfriend, the cheery ever-helpful manager who runs this place—has already left for the day or disappeared. This person before me is someone else.

"Who are you, then?"

A phantasm, another sort of angel in her same form—"I trust you'll be staying awhile longer with us."

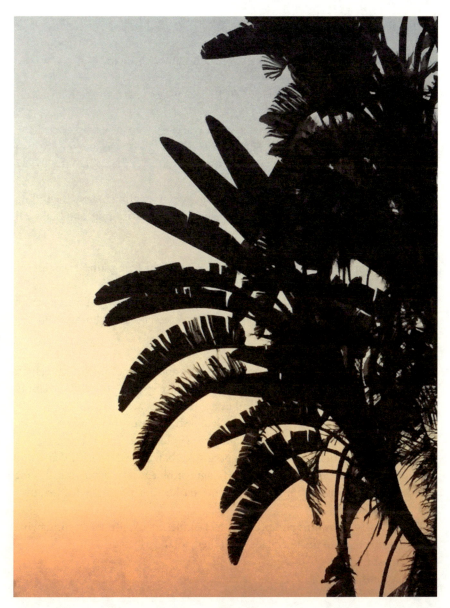
endings

Giggling nervously now, "No, I don't think I'm quite ready. I mean, I don't qualify."

"No, sweetie. None of them were ready at first. Most of them still aren't. And qualification isn't a problem, either. You know how things work here today"—forms, contracts, corruption?—"It's all part of God's plan. It just depends on the message I get from above about what you deserve and when you'll go. And not through the gate you came in today."

"Thanks again," I lurch. "More to come!"

Luckily, the waiting room's door is still open. It slams behind me on the way out.
"Sorry!"

I don't look back. Again, that fiery Old Testament story sears through me warning me not to.

Unlock, crank the parking break, grip the wheel—go, go for Christ's sake!

Down the driveway, past the darkened cottages—the travel nurses are also already gone for the day. Macadamia nuts are rolling all over the floor of the Toyota like shrapnel.

Pretty is still on duty in the guard house and sees us coming in hot. The sliding gate's opening just in time for the escape. She knows we're running, and that we'll never escape from what we are running from.

Suddenly, a rumbling—as the horizon clips the last of the dying sun, at the threshold between home and the real world,

The ground next to us unsettles. Dust falls beneath the cracks that scatter across the surface, turning the patches of scrub grass into desert islands. From within the widenings, sharp, hot light:

An explosion.

The wooden stakes, ignited, shrink to kindling and then nothing in an instant, and the once barren gravesite is entirely awash in fire spewing beyond the empty patch of lawn toward the driveway and underneath the car.

All around us, a white heat. Flames kick and shear the doors. The fire:

Blood reds, oranges, fire-hued, shimmering golds, the flashed cracking of a thousand peridot gem faces, new grassroots greens, banana leaf greens, *luhlaza lokwebhacabhaca*, that deep Zulu word for the green-blue where water and sky fade into one another, waves of purple iridescence flashed in a peacock's feather, dye-rich indigo. The smoke:

Black velvet-like swaths enrapturing the last flickers of light, of anything visibly remaining of us in the hot chaos. And then, total darkness:

A starless night-sky black,

The cosmos,

The end.

~

"Excuse me? Sir?"

A shiver,

And then pulled focus on the voice and woman standing in front of me. No magenta lips this time, but a blousy shirt, blue vest, and gold name tag with wings—a standard-issue uniform. Again though, I can smell cigarette smoke ema-

CONFESSIONS 195

nating from somewhere nearby. Probably the Wimpy restaurant's patio just beyond the sliding glass doors.

We survived,

And made it to the flight on time. It was all a dream—the end-of-shift end-times part at least. Another softened voice carries through the airwaves of the speaker system, announcing where the bags will end up, where the next flight leaves from— next to Cape Town, next to Johannesburg.

"Next? Sir?"

"Sorry." Still lost in memories for now. The where, how, and when this came to be is more than I can remember.

I look at my phone again while she processes my ticket. Instagram is all ads now, fewer posts from friends. In WhatsApp, two light-blue checkmarks show that Angel saw my last message asking her how things are going and about how all of this should wrap up, but there's still no response—"left on read" as the Millennials say. She's just busy as always, I tell myself.

I believe the map I started with got us to where we needed to be by the end—a place where we found grace or something else extraordinary, a miracle really since it was also out of the way and a lot of the places around here have multiple names—old ones, new ones. Again, confusion—we could've been lost. Or worse. A better map might combine or layer the old and new, bring together those who know each, to show we *can* coexist—rather than crowd each other out.

And yet, every place—every body—cannot be captured on a GPS map. Or security camera, for that matter.

I suddenly remember the taxi driver who brought me to the airport just now—a gray-bearded black man—mkhulu. Maybe he's husband or brother to that gogo who sold me the nuts this morning. Or he's actually Grandpa Malopa on a side hustle. (Once I read that almost a quarter of U.S. Uber drivers are over fifty-five.)

Mkhulu jokes that his name is Donald Trump.

"You know, it's not too late to turn around," I joke back, not wanting to return quite yet to the political mess at home. Still, I miss Charlie. Mom and Dad. Even the plants.

It must be 100 degrees today—almost 38 Celsius. Lush, hot. Sun blasting.

"Stay, baba," he chuckles. "We know where you belong. Stay and live your life for today. It is a present, remember. A gift from God."

Where do I belong? I wonder. Who's "we"?

I squint to see him in the glare of the taxi's rearview mirror but instead see myself. Fuzzy—I need a new glasses prescription, but I do catch sight of crow's feet, my own gray hairs.

I shudder.

(I never escaped. We never will.)

He winks. "Just remember to tip."

Acknowledgments

The research and writing for this book was made possible by the Wenner-Gren Foundation; the Reed Foundation's Ruth Landes Memorial Research Fund; the University of the Witwatersrand's (Wits) Research Council; and, from the University of New Hampshire, the Mellon Foundation–funded Global Racial and Social Inequality Lab, the Center for the Humanities through a Burnham Fellowship, a Faculty Fellowship, a Saul O. Sidore Memorial Lecture Series Award, and the Office of the Provost through a Faculty Scholars Award.

Besides the stars who shared their stories, many others deserve to be named for being cheerleaders, critical readers or research leads, fellow coffee shop writers, angels, and other extraordinary people among us: Liza Reniers, Katrien Botha, Crisma Zaayman, Razia Saleh, Christo Brand, Mzwandile Lukhele, Nolwazi Mkhwanazi, Lenore Manderson, Hylton White, Julia Hornberger, Sharad Chari, Danai Mupotsa, Sarah Duff, Shireen Hassim, Sarah Nuttall, Hlonipha Mokoena, Keith Breckenridge, Cath Burns, Rebecca Hodes, Fran Lisa Buntman, Jarred Thompson, M. Wolff, Charlotte Visagie, Tamia Botes, Maggie Davey, Roshan Cader, Bongani Ndodana-Breen, Charl Blignaut, Renugan Raidoo, Claudia Gastrow, Jessica Ruthven, Marissa Mika, Rosemarie Garland-Thomson, Ann Neumann, Eve Fairbanks, Kimberly Guinta, Carah Naseem, Sarah Lamb, Janet McIntosh, Julie Livingston, Noah Tamarkin, Todne Thomas, T. J. Tallie, Ieva Jusionyte, Anna Jaysane-Darr, Jessica Hardin, Anna Corwin, Jessica Robbins-Ruszkowski, Paul Wenzel Geissler, Cati Coe, Robin E. Sheriff, Siobhan Senier, Cristina Faiver-Serna, Daniel Callahan, Dayo Fadelu, and of course Ken and Monica Golomski and Charlie Favalora.

Over the years, I shared and workshopped this book with audiences at Wits Institute for Social and Economic Research (WISER) and Anthropology; the University of Pretoria; the University of Wisconsin; the University of Edinburgh and the University of Malawi's Wellcome Trust Medical and Health Humanities in Africa Workshop; Boston University; the Canadian Anthropological Society and American Anthropological Association meetings; the Northeastern Workshops on

Southern Africa; the University of Oslo; and the African Studies Workshop and the Weatherhead Center for International Affairs' Friday Morning Seminar in Culture, Psychiatry, and Global Mental Health at Harvard University.

At the University of New Hampshire (UNH), my colleagues in Anthropology and Women's and Gender Studies were unwavering supporters. My collaborations with colleagues in Social Work, the Center for Aging and Community Living, and Institute on Disability on public-facing research around aging, housing, and social services in the United States helped me to put much of this South African story in global perspective.

Thanks especially to friends and fora that engaged and encouraged my experiments in creative writing: editors at *Somatosphere*, *Annals of Global Health*, *Medical Humanities*, *Sheepshead Review*, and *The Gravity of the Thing*; the Society for Humanistic Anthropology Writing Awards and *Anthropology & Humanism*; Paul Wenzel Geissler and colleagues at the University of Oslo; Ieva Jusionyte and her student-colleagues, then at Harvard University; Nolwazi Mkhwanazi and her postdoctoral scholar-colleagues at the University of Pretoria; David Rivard and our fellow poets in the UNH MFA program; Alex Nading, Abby Neely, Laura Meek, and colleagues for conversing "beyond the limits" in *Medical Anthropology Quarterly*; Carole McGranahan and Sienna R. Craig and our fellow flash nonfiction writers; and Elizabeth E. Ferry, Caitrin Lynch, Sarah Pinto, and Steven Gonzalez of our Nashoba Writing Group. It all started there.

Portions of this book were previously published in *Anthropology & Aging* and *Africa* and are reprinted with permission.

Notes

PREFACE

1. Kirin Narayan, *Alive in the Writing: Crafting Ethnography in the Company of Chekhov* (Chicago: University of Chicago Press, 2012); Kirin Narayan, "Tools to Shape Texts: What Creative Nonfiction Can Offer Ethnography," *Anthropology and Humanism* 32, no. 2 (2007): 130–144. See also Helena Wulff, ed., *The Anthropologist as Writer: Genres and Contexts in the Twenty-First Century* (London: Berghahn Books, 2016); Carole McGranahan, ed., *Writing Anthropology: Essays on Craft and Commitment* (Durham, NC: Duke University Press, 2020). A few books that inspired me to write this one include Elissa Washuta, *White Magic* (New York: Tin House Books, 2021); Bongani Kona, ed., *Our Ghosts Were Once People: Stories on Death and Dying* (Cape Town: Jonathan Ball, 2021); Todd Meyers, *All That Was Not Her* (Durham, NC: Duke University Press, 2021); Zora Neale Hurston, *Barracoon: The Story of the Last "Black Cargo"* (New York: Amistad Books, 2018); Theresa Brown, *The Shift: One Nurse, Twelve Hours, Four Patients' Lives* (Chapel Hill, NC: Algonquin Books, 2015); Renato Rosaldo, *The Day of Shelly's Death: The Poetry and Ethnography of Grief* (Durham, NC: Duke University Press, 2014); and the writing of vangile gantsho, Zakes Mda, Yannis Ritsos, and Wisława Szymborska.

2. On Freud and Melanie Klein's notions of superego in critical and cross-cultural perspective, see Jennifer Yusin, *The Future Life of Trauma: Partitions, Borders, Repetition* (New York: Fordham University Press, 2017); J. Lorand Matory, *The Fetish Revisited: Marx, Freud, and the Gods Black People Make* (Durham, NC: Duke University Press, 2018); Terry Eagleton, *Radical Sacrifice* (New Haven, CT: Yale University Press, 2018). Nadira Omarjee argues that each time we critically confront our superego as a form of our society's values, we can undo or decolonize a previous sense of ourselves and generate new values to change prevailing systems for a better world. Nadira Omarjee, *We Belong to the Earth: Towards a Decolonial Feminist Pedagogy Rooted in Uhuru and Ubuntu* (Bamenda, Cameroon: Langaa RPCIG, 2023), 23.

3. Lars Tornstam, *Gerotranscendence: A Developmental Theory of Positive Aging* (New York: Springer, 2005); Erik S. Wortman and Jordan P. Lewis, "Gerotranscendence and Alaska Native Successful Aging in the Aleutian Pribilof Islands, Alaska," *Journal of Cross-Cultural Gerontology* 36, no. 1 (2021): 43–67; Doris Bohman, Neltjie C. van Wyk, and Sirkka-Liisa Ekman, "South Africans' Experience of Being Old and of Care and Caring in a Transitional Period," *International Journal of Older People Nursing* 6, no. 3 (2010): 187–195; Jason Danely, "Hope in an Aging Japan," *Contemporary Japan* 28, no. 1 (2016): 13–31; Anna I. Corwin, *Embracing Age: How Catholic Nuns Become Models for Aging Well* (New Brunswick, NJ: Rutgers University Press, 2021).

4. Kevin Gaines, *Black Expatriates and the Civil Rights Era: American Africans in Ghana* (Chapel Hill: University of North Carolina Press, 2006); Robert T. Vinson, *The Americans*

Are Coming! Dreams of African American Liberation in Segregationist South Africa (Athens: Ohio University Press, 2012); Tanisha Ford, *Liberated Threads: Black Women, Style, and the Global Politics of Soul* (Chapel Hill: University of North Carolina Press, 2015); Lisa Brock, Van Gosse, and Alex Lichtenstein, eds., "The Global Antiapartheid Movement: Editors' Introduction," special issue, *Radical History Review* 14, no. 2 (2014); Keisha Blain and Tiffany Gill, eds., *Turn the Whole World Over: Black Women and Internationalism* (Champaign: University of Illinois Press, 2019); Lyn Ossome, Athinangamso Esther Nkopo, and Danai S. Mupotsa, eds., "Black Transnational Feminisms and the Question of Structure," special issue, *Agenda* 36, no. 4 (2022); and biographies of black women engaged in transnational activism like Lillian Ngoyi, Florence Moposho, Audre Lorde, and Angela Davis. In South Africa, many citizens who self-identify as coloured—itself a racial category that emerged amid European colonization and persists today—engage blackness as part of their commitments to African feminisms, nonracialism, black consciousness, and or Pan-Africanism. See Zmitri Erasmus, *Coloured by History, Shaped by Place: New Perspectives on Coloured Identities in Cape Town* (Cape Town: Kwela, 2001); Whitney N. Laster Pirtle, "Racial Identity Choices among 'Coloureds' as Shaped by the South African Racial State," *Identities* 30, no. 3 (2023): 392–410. "White" as a racial identity in this book remains in lower case as well, to avoid signal boosting or yoking individuals to its overtly supremacist formations.

5. One aspect of this creative writing process is balancing fidelity, or faithfulness to what happened "in the moment," and partial reinventions in retelling what happened "after the fact." Expanding on the long-standing critiques by George Marcus, James Clifford, and others of ethnographic "truth" and objectivity, Angela Garcia notes that "invention runs the risk of obscuring this fidelity (although this is not necessarily a bad thing). Other times, invention succeeds in unsettling and expanding the limit of what can be seen and felt, changing the terms upon which fidelity is rendered and understood." Angela Garcia, "Fidelity and Invention," in *Crumpled Paper Boat: Experiments in Ethnographic Writing*, ed. Anand Pandian and Stuart McLean (Durham, NC: Duke University Press, 2017), 223.

6. Over the span of seven years, I was vetted by three institutional review boards—the University of Massachusetts Boston, the University of New Hampshire, and the University of the Witwatersrand—to conduct ethical research with the home's staff and residents, receiving permission (informed written and or verbal consent) by residents, staff, and the home's manager on behalf of the home's larger organization. I also shared drafts of chapters with featured individuals for feedback which I then incorporated.

7. Anne Dufourmantelle, *Power of Gentleness: Meditations on the Risk of Living*, trans. Katherine Payne and Vincent Sallé (New York: Fordham University Press, 2018); Casey Golomski, "Gentleness," *Medical Anthropology Quarterly* 37, no. 2 (2023): 98–101. See the last chapter of this book, "Confessions," for more on grace.

THE ROAD

1. Channing Hargrove, "Why Did Etsy Shut Down This 'Pro-Black, Anti-Bullshit' Shop?," *Refinery29*, September 12, 2018.

2. Fran Baum et al., "New Perspective on Why Women Live Longer Than Men: An Exploration of Power, Gender, Social Determinants, and Capitals," *International Journal of Environmental Research and Public Health* 18, no. 2 (January 14, 2021): 661.

3. Ashon Crawley, "Otherwise Movements," *The New Inquiry*, January 18, 2015; Tiffany Lethabo King, Jenell Navarro, and Andrew Smith, eds., *Otherwise Worlds: Against Settler Colonialism and Anti-Blackness* (Durham, NC: Duke University Press, 2020); Samuel Huard, "The Otherwise and Grace: Exploring Theopolitical Connections," *Studies in Religion/Sciences Religieuses* (December 9, 2023), doi: 10.1177/00084298231212200.

4. Nelson Mandela, *Long Walk to Freedom* (Boston: Little, Brown, 1994).

WAITING

1. Thando Mgqolozana, *A Man Who Is Not a Man* (Scottsville: University of KwaZulu-Natal Press, 2009); Gcobani Qambela, "'The Boy Has to Be a Man in Order for Life to Start':

NOTES TO PAGES 7–10

AmaXhosa, Black Boyhood Studies, and the Anthropology of Boyhoods," *South African Review of Sociology* 52, no. 2 (2022): 40–56.

2. Thomas C. Buchmueller et al., "Effect of the Affordable Care Act on Racial and Ethnic Disparities in Health Insurance Coverage," *American Journal of Public Health* 106, no. 8 (2016): 1416–1421.

3. Jim Rutenberg and Jackie Calmes, "False Death Panel Has Some Familiar Rumors," *New York Times*, August 14, 2009; Allyson Coldiron et al., "Older Adults' Persisting Beliefs about the Death Panel Myth and Advance Directives," *Innovation in Aging* 4, suppl. 1 (2020): 68.

4. Kirsten J. Colello, *The Elder Justice Act: Background and Issues for Congress*, Congressional Research Service Report No. R43707, June 15, 2020.

5. Jonathan Metzl, *Dying of Whiteness: How Racial Resentment Is Killing America's Heartland* (New York: Basic Books, 2019).

6. Robert van Niekerk, "Healthy Policy Reform in the Last Days of Apartheid and the Dilemmas Facing the ANC," in *Universal Health Care in Southern Africa: Policy Contestation in Health System Reform in South Africa and Zimbabwe*, ed. Greg Ruiters and Robert van Niekerk (Scottsville: University of KwaZulu-Natal Press, 2012), 55–64.

7. Caryn Bredenkamp et al., "Changing Inequalities in Health-Adjusted Life Expectancy by Income and Race in South Africa," *Health Systems & Reform* 7, no. 2 (2021): e1909303.

8. R. E. Dorrington et al., "The Impact of the SARS-CoV-2 Epidemic on Mortality in South Africa in 2020," *South African Medical Journal* 112, no. 1 (2022): 14–16.

9. Casey Golomski, "Elder Care and Private Health Insurance in South Africa: The Pathos of Race-Class," *Medical Anthropology* 37, no. 4 (2018): 311–326.

10. Silke van Dyk and Thomas Küpper, eds., "Theorizing Age—Postcolonial Perspectives in Aging Studies," special issue, *Journal of Aging Studies* 39 (2016); Terrell D. Brown and KenZoe Brian J. Selassie, "From These Roots: The Role of Historically Black Colleges and Universities in Preparing the Nation's Gerontologists for an Aging Society," *Journal of Human Behavior in the Social Environment* 27, no. 5 (2017): 385–393; Sweta Rajan-Rankin, "Race, Embodiment and Later Life: Re-Animating Aging Bodies of Color," *Journal of Aging Studies* 45 (2018): 32–38; Molly George, *Aging in a Changing World: Older New Zealanders and Contemporary Multiculturalism* (New Brunswick, NJ: Rutgers University Press, 2021); Saloua Berdai Chaouni et al., "Doing Research on the Intersection of Ethnicity and Old Age: Key Insights from Decolonial Frameworks," *Journal of Aging Studies* 56 (2021): 100909; Sandra Torres, "Racialization and Racism," in *Handbook of Migration and Ageing*, ed. Sandra Torres and Alistair Hunter (Northampton, MA: Edward Elgar, 2023), 107–117; Metzl, *Dying of Whiteness*.

11. National Center for Health Statistics, *Biennial Overview of Post-Acute and Long-Term Care in the United States: Data from the 2020 National Post-Acute and Long-Term Care Study* (Atlanta: Centers for Disease Control and Prevention), last updated September 26, 2023, https://www.cdc.gov/nchs/npals/webtables/overview.htm. This figure total combines residential care (30,600 facilities and 818,800 users) and certified nursing homes (15,300 facilities and 1,294,800 users), excluding home health agencies, in-patient rehab facilities, long-term care hospitals, and hospice. Hospice serves many older adults, mostly for neurological conditions like Alzheimer's, but it varies as to location of its care application and users' comparatively shorter stays versus stays in residential-type hospice settings. See also National Hospice and Palliative Care Organization, *NHPCO Facts and Figures 2023 Edition*, December 2023.

12. Roxanne Jacobs et al., *The Impact of Covid-19 on Long-Term Care Facilities in South Africa with a Specific Focus on Dementia Care*, STRiDE / International Long-Term Care Policy Network, 2020, 9.

13. Carnegie Commission of Investigation on the Poor White Question in South Africa, *The Poor White Problem in South Africa: Report of the Carnegie Commission* (Stellenbosch, Western Cape: Pro Ecclesia-Drukkery, 1932); Tiffany Willoughby-Herard. *Waste of a White Skin: The Carnegie Corporation and the Racial Logic of White Vulnerability* (Berkeley: University of California Press, 2015).

14. Marijke du Toit, "Women, Welfare and the Nurturing of Afrikaner Nationalism: A Social History of the Afrikaanse Christelike Vroue Vereniging, c. 1870–1939" (PhD diss.,

University of Cape Town, 1996); Charl Blignaut, "'Die Hand Aan Die Wieg Regeer Die Land' [The Hand That Rocks the Cradle Rules the Land]: Exploring the Agency and Identity of Women in the Ossewa-Brandwag, 1939–1954," *South African Historical Journal* 67, no. 1 (2015): 47–63.

15. Andreas Sagner, "Ageing and Social Policy in South Africa," *Journal of Southern African Studies* 26, no. 3 (2002): 523–553.

16. Shireen Ally and Arianna Lissoni, eds., *New Histories of South Africa's Apartheid-Era Bantustans* (New York: Routledge, 2017).

17. See Department of Coloured Affairs, Union of South Africa, *Report of the Department of Coloured Affairs for the Period 1st April, 1955, to 31st December, 1958*, UG No. 32/1960 (Pretoria: Government Printer, 1960); Department of Health and Social Services, Bophuthatswana (South Africa), *Annual Report*, 1980, 1983, 1989, in African Government Documents, African Studies Library, Boston University; Department of Health and Social Welfare, Gazankulu (South Africa), *Annual Report*, 1984–1985, 1989–1990, in African Government Documents, African Studies Library, Boston University. For example, nearly fifteen years after its establishment, Gazankulu's administrators noted that "geriatric nursing services" "are nonexistent in a collective institutionalised and organized pattern" in their homeland, and that it needed "urgent organization of special geriatric health and welfare services to the benefit of the aged and the student nurse who must have a broad and collective view of the total health needs of our old citizens" (Department of Health and Social Welfare, Gazankulu (South Africa), *Annual Report*, 1984–1985, 36–37). The inaugural report for the homeland of Bophuthatswana recorded 40,042 old age pensioners, 6,537 of whom also received a disability and leprosy pension and 1,600 of whom also received a pension for the blind, as well as three old age homes "operated by missions or private bodies but financed by Government" that housed 269 people. Bophuthatswana Government (South Africa), *Bophuthatswana at Independence, 6 December 1977* (Pretoria: Bureau for Economic Research re Bantu Development, 1977), 21–22.

18. Franco Frescura, "Designing for a Developing Economy," *Building*, April 19, 1989, 11–15; "Nhlumba Bertha Mkhize," *South Africa History Online*, last updated November 19, 2020; Mbali Mkhize, personal communication courtesy of Meghan Healy-Clancy, February 28, 2024.

19. Cape Party-Kaapse Party v. Iziko South African National Gallery, EC 02/2017 (Cape Town: Equality Court, Magistrates' Court, Cape Town).

20. Karen Gonsalkorale, Jeffrey W. Sherman, and Karl Christoph Klauer, "Aging and Prejudice: Diminished Regulation of Automatic Race Bias among Older Adults," *Journal of Experimental Social Psychology* 45, no. 2 (2009): 410–414; Robby Berman, "Wait. Is Grandma a Racist?," *Big Think*, July 8, 2018.

21. Metzl, *Dying of Whiteness*; Patrik Marier and Marina Revelli, "Compassionate Canadians and Conflictual Americans? Portrayals of Ageism in Liberal and Conservative Media," *Ageing and Society* 37, no. 8 (2017): 1632–1653; Kevin Munger, *Generation Gap: Why the Baby Boomers Still Dominate American Politics and Culture* (New York: Columbia University Press, 2022).

22. Margaret Morganroth Gullette, *Ending Ageism, or How Not to Shoot Old People* (New Brunswick, NJ: Rutgers University Press, 2017); Jennifer Sawyer et al., "When Grandpa Says Something Racist: The Role of Ageism in Young Adult Responses," *Innovation in Aging* 3, suppl. 1 (2019): S82; George, *Aging in a Changing World*.

23. The aging prison population in the United States is steadily rising, and by age fifty many individuals who are incarcerated long-term are categorized as physically "elderly" as the prison environment destroys their bodies so quickly. Compassionate release policies exist that would permit parole or leave for nondangerous, aging, ill, and dying incarcerated people, but such policies are rarely used. See the Release Aging People in Prison Campaign and Emily Widra, "The Aging Prison Population: Causes, Costs, and Consequences," *The Prison Policy Initiative*, August 2, 2023.

24. Bredenkamp et al., "Changing Inequalities"; Hannes Schwandt et al., "Inequality in Mortality between Black and White Americans by Age, Place, and Cause and in Comparison to Europe, 1990 to 2018," *PNAS* 118, no. 40 (2021): e2104681118; Metzl, *Dying of Whiteness*.

NOTES TO PAGES 14–22

25. Andrew Lawrence, "Uju Anya on the Queen, Jeff Bezos and the Family History behind Her Tweet," *Guardian*, September 14, 2022; D. L. Chandler, "Black Twitter and Irish Twitter Cook Prince Philip after News of Passing," *Hip Hop Wired*, April 9, 2021; Barnor Hesse, "Racialized Modernity: An Analytic of White Mythologies," *Ethnic and Racial Studies* 30, no. 4 (2007): 643–663.

26. Janet McIntosh, *Unsettled: Denial and Belonging among White Kenyans* (Berkeley: University of California Press, 2016); Nicky Falkof, *The End of Whiteness: Satanism and Family Murder in Late Apartheid South Africa* (Auckland Park: Jacana Media, 2016); Derek Hook, "White Anxiety in (Post)Apartheid South Africa," *Psychoanalysis, Culture & Society* 25 (2020): 612–631; Scott Burnett, *White Belongings: Race, Land, and Property in Post-Apartheid South Africa* (Lanham, MD: Lexington Books, 2022).

27. For example, the mass shooting at Tops Friendly Markets in Buffalo, NY, May 2022, among many others. See also Cassie Miller, "SPLC Poll Finds Substantial Support for 'Great Replacement' Theory and Other Hard-Right Ideas," Southern Poverty Law Center, June 1, 2022; Barnor Hesse, "Black Populism," *Southern Atlantic Quarterly* 121, no. 3 (2022): 561–592.

28. Vincent Crapanzano, *Waiting: The Whites of South Africa* (New York: Random House, 1986), 45.

29. J. M. Coetzee, "Listening to the Afrikaners," *New York Times*, April 14, 1985.

30. J. M. Coetzee, *Age of Iron: A Novel* (London: Secker and Warburg, 1990), 197.

31. Craig Higginson. *The Dream House: A Novel* (Johannesburg: Picador Africa, 2015), viii.

32. Gullette, *Ending Ageism*.

33. Higginson, *Dream House*, x.

34. Yewande Omotoso, *The Woman Next Door* (Johannesburg: Picador Africa, 2017). See also Futhi Ntshingila, *They Got to You Too: A Novel* (Northampton, MA: Interlink Books, 2023).

35. Jacobs et al., *Impact of Covid-19*; A. Perold and Marie Muller, "The Composition of Old Age Homes in South Africa in Relation to the Residents and Nursing Personnel," *Curationis* (March 2020): 87–94; Lesego M. Ramocha, Quinette A. Louw, and Muziwakhe D. Tshabalala, "Quality of Life and Physical Activity among Older Adults Living in Institutions Compared to the Community," *South African Journal of Physiotherapy* 73, no. 1 (2017): a342; Jessica Ruthven, "Suffering Grannies," in *Connected Lives: Families, Households, Health and Care in Contemporary South Africa*, ed. Nolwazi Mkhwanazi and Lenore Manderson (Cape Town: Human Sciences Research Council, 2020), 180–185.

36. Timothy Bates, Ginachukwu Amah, and Janet Coffman, *Racial/Ethnic Diversity in the Long-Term Care Workforce* (San Francisco: Health Workforce Research Center on Long-Term Care, University of California San Francisco, 2018); Cati Coe, *The New American Servitude: Political Belonging among African Immigrant Home Care Workers* (New York: New York University Press, 2017).

ANGEL

1. Unless cited otherwise, all quoted monetary figures in rand (ZAR) represent stated cost and USD conversion at the time of a respective interview. Across the entire period of field research, January 1, 2015, to September 30, 2022, the conversion rate for USD 1.00 rose steadily from ZAR 11.64 to just over ZAR 18.00. Query the International Monetary Fund Exchange Rate Report Wizard, using representative exchange rates for South Africa and the United States with the above dates for further details.

2. Peter Lloyd-Sherlock and S. Agrawal, "Pensions and the Health of Older People in South Africa: Is There an Effect?," *Journal of Development Studies* 50, no. 11 (2014): 1570–1586; Guy Harling et al., "Impairment in Activities of Daily Living, Care Receipt, and Unmet Needs in a Middle-Aged and Older Rural South African Population: Findings from the HAALSI Study," *Journal of Aging and Health* 32, nos. 5–6 (2020): 296–307; Carlos Ruimallo Herl et al., "Pension Exposure and Health: Evidence from a Longitudinal Study in South Africa," *Journal of Ageing and Economics* 23 (2022): 10411; James Ferguson, *Give a Man a Fish: Reflections on the New Politics of Distribution* (Durham, NC: Duke University Press, 2015).

3. "Old Age Pension," South African Government Official Information and Services, accessed May 4, 2024, https://www.gov.za/services/services-residents/social-benefits/old-age -pension.

4. Daniel Steyn, "Old Age Grant Is Not Enough to Cover Care Needs, Researchers Find," GroundUp, February 15, 2024.

5. Nicoli Nattrass and Jeremy Seekings, "'Two Nations'? Race and Economic Inequality in South Africa Today," *Daedalus* 130, no. 1 (2001): 45–70; Statistics South Africa, *Inequality Trends in South Africa: A Multidimensional Diagnostic of Inequality*, Report 03-10-19 (Pretoria: Statistics South Africa, 2019); Victor Sulla, Precious Zikhali, and Pablo Facundo Cuevas, *Inequality in Southern Africa: An Assessment of the Southern African Customs Union (English)* (Washington, DC: World Bank Group, 2022).

6. Natasha Thandiwe Vally, "Insecurity in South African Social Security: An Examination of Social Grant Deductions, Cancellations, and Waiting," *Journal of Southern African Studies* 42, no. 5 (2016): 965–982; Department of Home Affairs, South African Government, "Minister Malusi Gigaba: Progress in the War on Queues Campaign and Resignation of the Director-General," media release, July 23, 2018; Steve Kretzmann, "Queue, the Beloved Country: Welcome to Aaron Motsoaledi's Dysfunctional Department of Home Affairs," *Daily Maverick*, May 14, 2022.

7. Deborah James, *Money from Nothing: Indebtedness and Aspiration in South Africa* (Redwood City, CA: Stanford University Press, 2014).

8. Dineo Skosana, "Grave Matters: Dispossession and the Desecration of Ancestral Graves by Mining Corporations in South Africa," *Journal of Contemporary African Studies* 40, no. 1 (2022): 47–62.

9. Along with English, most of the residents and management team at Grace spoke Afrikaans. I struggled to learn it, and in September 2019, the incredibly talented researcher Tamia Botes assisted me for a week in participant observation and conversation-based research with Afrikaans-speaking residents. Later, Charlotte Visagie assisted me in translating some of the home's historic correspondence from Afrikaans to English.

10. I learned isiZulu and siSwati through the U.S. Title 7 language programs at Boston University's Center for African Studies; a U.S. Fulbright-Hays Group Project Abroad in Intermediate-Advanced isiZulu through the University of KwaZulu-Natal, Pietermartizburg; and by talking with many Southern African people over many years. See Casey Golomski, *Funeral Culture: AIDS, Work and Cultural Change in an African Kingdom* (Bloomington: Indiana University Press, 2018). Historically, the siSwati language and liSwati ethnicity were called "Swazi," and the British Protectorate-then-country of Swaziland changed its name to eSwatini in 2018. In this book, I use "Swazi" only when in reference to specific historical contexts or when directly quoting a source where it's used.

11. AbdouMaliq Simone, "People as Infrastructure: Intersecting Fragments in Johannesburg," *Public Culture* 16, no. 3 (2004): 407–429; Pumla Gqola, "Race and/as the Rainbow Nation Nightmare," paper presented at the Public Positions on History and Politics Seminar, Wits University, Johannesburg, 2015; Grace Musila, "Laughing at the Rainbow's Cracks? Blackness, Whiteness and the Ambivalence of South African Stand-Up Comedy," in *Civic Agency in Africa: Arts of Resistance in the 21st Century*, ed. Ebenezer Obadare and W. Willems (Suffolk, UK: James Currey, 2014), 147–166; April Sizemore Barber, *Prismatic Performances: Queer South Africa and the Fragmentation of the Rainbow Nation* (Ann Arbor: University of Michigan Press, 2020).

12. Alan Mabin, "A Century of South African Housing Acts 1920–2020," *Urban Forum* 31 (2020): 453–472.

13. Laurine Platzky and Cherryl Walker, *The Surplus People: Forced Removals in South Africa* (Johannesburg: Ravan Press, 1985).

14. Robina Goodlad, "The Housing Challenge in South Africa," *Urban Studies* 33, no. 9 (1996): 1629–1645.

15. Ashwin Desai, *We Are the Poors* (New York: Monthly Review Press, 2002); Kerry Chance, *Living Politics in South Africa's Urban Shacklands* (Chicago: University of Chicago Press, 2017); Gaster Sharpley, "Government Housing Rectification Program and Practice in South Africa" (PhD diss., University of the Western Cape, 2018).

NOTES TO PAGES 28–59

16. In isiMpondo and other languages, *ukwakumkanya* means "creating a shadow in order to illuminate" and critically much more as part of critical black perspectives on the world. See Hugo ka Canham, *Riotous Deathscapes* (Durham, NC: Duke University Press, 2023).

17. A gendered term for the home's organizational headquarters.

18. "Nelspruit the Segregated City," South African History Online, accessed March 23, 2023, https://www.sahistory.org.za/article/nelspruit-segregated-city.

19. Waasila Jassat et al., "The Intersection of Age, Sex, Race and Socioeconomic Status in COVID-19 Hospital Admissions and Deaths in South Africa," *South African Journal of Science* 118, nos. 5–6 (2022): 1–14.

PRESENTS

1. Ilana van Wyk, "'Tata ma Chance': On Contingency and the Lottery in Postapartheid South Africa," *Africa* 82, no. 1 (2012): 41–68.

2. "Information," Powerball.net, accessed March 23, 2023; Christine Hobden, "Is It Time to Stop Buying That Powerball Ticket?," *Daily Maverick*, March 8, 2022.

3. "Baas" means "boss" in Afrikaans and registers inequalities between white employers and black workers. See Oswald Mbuyiseni Mtshali's poem "The Watchman's Blues" in his collection *Song of the Cowhide Drum* (New York: Third Press, 1972), 50.

4. Zolani Ngwane, "'Christmas Time' and the Struggles for the Household in the Countryside: Rethinking the Cultural Geography of Migrant Labour in South Africa," *Journal of Southern African Studies* 29, no. 3 (2003): 681–699.

5. For a critical interpretation, see Casey Golomski, "'Yesterday Is History, Tomorrow Is a Mystery': Dying in South African Frail Care," *Anthropology & Aging* 41, no. 2 (2020): 9–23.

6. "No Name Change for Rhodes University Following Council Vote," *Mail and Guardian*, December 6, 2017.

7. Nhlanhla Ndebele and Noor Nieftagodien, "The Morogoro Conference: A Moment of Self-Reflection," in *The Road to Democracy in South Africa*, vol. 1, *1960–1970*, ed. South African Democracy Education Trust (Cape Town: Struik, 2005), 573–599.

8. Hugh MacMillan, *Chris Hani* (Auckland Park, Johannesburg: Jacana, 2014).

9. Bernadette Wicks, "Fraser Overruled Only One Negative Recommendation for Medical Parole—Zuma's," *EWN*, November 21, 2022.

10. Rédaction Africanews with AFP, "Anti-Apartheid Icon Chris Hani's Grave Vandalized," *Africanews*, November 29, 2022.

11. The White House, "Cheaper Hearing Aids Now in Stores Thanks to Biden-Harris Administration Competition Agenda," fact sheet, October 17, 2022.

ANDREW

1. Michael Schulman, "Is There a 'Gay Voice?,'" *New Yorker*, July 10, 2015; Fabio Fasoli, Peter Hegarty, and David M. Frost, "Stigmatization of 'Gay-Sounding' Voices: The Role of Heterosexual, Lesbian, and Gay Individuals' Essentialist Beliefs," *British Journal of Social Psychology* 60, no. 3 (2021): 826–850.

2. Casey Golomski, "Countermythologies: Queering Lives in a Southern African Gay and Lesbian Pentecostal Church," *Transforming Anthropology* 28, no. 2 (2020): 155–168.

3. Keith Gardiner, ed., *Benoni: A Golden Anniversary for a Golden City* (self-pub., Henry Norval), 19, accessed March 23, 2023, lavrontech.co.za/Benoni/Benoni-History-23.pdf.

4. Michael W. Yarbrough, "Something Old, Something New: Historicizing Same-Sex Marriage within Ongoing Struggles over African Marriage in South Africa," *Sexualities* 21, no. 7 (2018): 1092–1108.

5. John Higginson, "Privileging the Machines: American Engineers, Indentured Chinese and White Workers in South Africa's Deep-Level Gold Mines, 1902–1907," *International Review of Social History* 52, no. 1 (2007): 1–34; Mae Ngai, *The Chinese Question: The Gold Rushes and Global Politics* (New York: W. W. Norton, 2021).

6. Jolene Marriah-Maharaj, "Teacher in Court over the Rape of Two Matric Pupils and the Impregnation of Both," *IOL News*, October 27, 2022; Lwazi Hlangu, "Durban Teacher

Accused of Raping Pupils Wants Bail Because He Has 'Diabetes, Migraines and Dependents,'" *DispatchLIVE*, May 4, 2022; Pumla Gqola, *Rape: A South African Nightmare* (Auckland Park, Johannesburg: Jacana, 2015).

7. Neil Henderson and Jamil Khan, "'I Will Die if I Have to Go into an Old Age Home': Afrocentric Options for Care of Older LGBT People in South Africa," *Agenda* 34, no. 1 (2020): 94–107; Linda Mkhize, "'And in Those Days to Be Gay Was Not On': Narratives of Older LGBT+ People in South Africa" (MA thesis, University of the Witwatersrand, 2022); Finn Reygan and Jamil Khan, "Sexual and Gender Diversity, Ageing and Elder Care in South Africa: Voices and Realities," in *Intersections of Ageing, Gender and Sexualities: Multidisciplinary International Perspectives*, ed. Andrew King, Kathryn Almack, and Rebecca L. Jones (Bristol, UK: Policy Press, 2019), 171–185.

8. Henderson and Khan, "I Will Die."

9. Reygan and Kahn, "Sexual and Gender Diversity."

10. LGBTQ Senior Housing, Inc., "The Pryde," accessed January 10, 2024, https://www.lgbtqseniorhousing.org/the-pryde.

11. Susannah Sudborough, "Hyde Park LGBTQ-Friendly Senior Housing Project Vandalized with Hate Speech," Boston.com, July 10, 2022, https://www.boston.com/news/local-news/2022/07/10/hyde-park-lgbtq-senior-housing-pryde-vandalized-hate-speech/.

12. Craig Seymour, cited in Spencer Kornhaber, "The Problem with Saying *Oontz Oontz*," *Atlantic*, July 28, 2022.

DIVERSITY

1. Melissa Steyn, *Whiteness Just Isn't What It Used to Be: White Identity in a Changing South Africa* (Albany: State University of New York Press, 2001).

2. Wits Centre for Diversity Studies, "DST-NRF SARChI Chair," University of the Witwatersrand, Johannesburg, accessed January 10, 2024, https://www.wits.ac.za/wicds/sarchi-chair/.

3. Pumla Gqola, *Rape: A South African Nightmare* (Auckland Park, Johannesburg: Jacana, 2015).

4. *The State. v. T. Makwanyane and M. Mchunu* (CCT3/94) [1995] ZACC 3; 1995 (6) BCLR 665; 1995 (3) SA 391; [1996] 2 CHRLD 164; 1995 (2) SACR 1 (Constitutional Court of the Republic of South Africa, June 6, 1995).

5. Tembeka Ngcukaitobi, *Land Matters: South Africa's Failed Land Reforms and the Road Ahead* (Pretoria: Penguin, 2021).

6. Andries du Toit, "The Land and Its People: The South African 'Land Question' and the Post-Apartheid Political Order" (PLAAS Working Paper No. 64, University of the Western Cape, March 2023).

BETHAL

1. Martha Webber, "Crafting Citizens: Material Rhetoric, Cultural Intermediaries, and the Amazwi Abesifazane South African National Quilt Project" (PhD diss., University of Illinois Urbana-Champaign, 2013).

2. Niq Mhlongo, ed., *Black Tax: Burden or Ubuntu* (Cape Town: Jonathan Ball, 2019).

3. Cati Coe, *The New American Servitude: Political Belonging among African Immigrant Home Care Workers* (New York: New York University Press, 2017); Katherine Nasol and Valerie Francisco-Menchavez, "Filipino Home Care Workers: Invisible Frontline Workers in the COVID-19 Crisis in the United States," *American Behavioral Scientist* 65, no. 10 (2021): 1365–1383; Lisa Dodson and Rebekah M. Zincavage, "'It's Like a Family': Caring Labor, Exploitation, and Race in Nursing Homes," *Gender & Society* 21, no. 6 (2007): 905–928; April Verrett, "Home Care Workers Are Now Called Essential," *Time*, August 24, 2020.

4. Leo Mapira, Gabrielle Kelly, and Leon N. Geffen, "A Qualitative Examination of Policy and Structural Factors Driving Care Workers' Adverse Experiences in Long-Term Residential Care Facilities for Older Adults in Cape Town," *BMC Geriatrics* 19, no. 97 (2019).

NOTES TO PAGES 78–99

5. Dodson and Zincavage, "'Like a Family'"; Coe, *New American Servitude.*

6. Aghogho Akpome, "Discourses of Corruption in Africa: Between the Colonial Past and the Decolonizing Present," *Africa Today* 67, no. 4 (2021): 10–29; Sapana Doshi and Malini Ranganathan, "Towards a Critical Geography of Corruption and Power in Late Capitalism," *Progress in Human Geography* 43, no. 3 (2019): 436–457.

7. Ben Farmer and Peta Thornycroft, "Mystery of Murdered Whistleblower Who Uncovered Hospital Corruption," *Telegraph*, October 11, 2022; Laetitia C. Rispel, Pieter de Jager, and Sharon Fonn, "Exploring Corruption in the South African Health Sector," *Health Policy and Planning* 31, no. 2 (2016): 239–249.

8. Jean Lee, "Travel Nurses' Gold Rush Is Over," NBC News, September 3, 2022.

9. April Hansen and Carol Tuttas, "Professional Choice 2020–2021: Travel Nursing Turns the Tide," *Nurse Leader* 20, no. 2 (2022): 145–151; April Hansen and Carol Tuttas, "Lived Travel Nurse and Permanent Staff Nurse Pandemic Work Experiences as Influencers of Motivation, Happiness, Stress, and Career Decisions," *Nursing Administration Quarterly* 46, no. 3 (2022): 245–254; Sydney Lake, "Travel Nurse Salaries Float around $200k as Staffing Crisis Continues," *Fortune*, November 17, 2022.

SAFARI

1. Jacob Dlamini, *Safari Nation: A Social History of the Kruger National Park* (Auckland Park, Johannesburg: Jacana, 2020).

2. Katy Tur and Henry Austin, "Lion Attack: U.S. Tourist Katherine Chappell Worked on 'Game of Thrones,'" NBC News, June 3, 2015.

3. Bongani Kona, "The Circle Will Not Be Unbound," in *Black Tax: Burden or Ubuntu?*, ed. Niq Mhlongo (Johannesburg: Jonathan Ball, 2019), 121–131.

4. Kona, "Circle Will Not Be Unbound," 130.

5. Braai means to barbeque.

GOODNESS

1. The verse from Matthew she refers to reads: "For I myself am a man under authority, with soldiers under me. I tell this one, 'Go,' and he goes; and that one, 'Come,' and he comes. I say to my servant, 'Do this,' and he does it" (New International Version).

2. CD4 count refers to a test to measure the number of CD4, a type of white blood cell, per cubic millimeter of blood. A normal CD4 range for healthy adults and teens is 500–1,200. For someone living with HIV, fewer than 500 indicates weakened immunity, and 200 or fewer is a threshold for an AIDS diagnosis.

3. Isak Niehaus, Eliazaar Mohlale, and Kally Shokane, *Witchcraft, Power and Politics: Exploring the Occult in the South African Lowveld* (London: Pluto Press, 2001), 147.

4. Niehaus, Mohlale, and Shokane, *Witchcraft, Power and Politics*; Birgit Meyer, *Translating the Devil: Religion and Modernity among the Ewe in Ghana* (Edinburgh: Edinburgh University Press, 1999); Brian Levack, ed., *The Oxford Handbook of Witchcraft in Early Modern Europe and Colonial America* (Oxford: Oxford University Press, 2015); Irene Silverblatt, *Sun, Moon and Witches: Gender Ideologies and Class in Inca and Colonial Peru* (Princeton, NJ: Princeton University Press, 1987).

5. Niehaus, Mohlale, and Shokane, *Witchcraft, Power and Politics*; Isak Niehaus, "From Witch-Hunts to Thief-Hunts: On the Temporality of Evil in South Africa," *African Historical Review* 44, no. 1 (2012): 29–52; Isak Niehaus, *Witchcraft and a Life in the New South Africa* (Cambridge: Cambridge University Press, 2013); Isak Niehaus, "Witches and Zombies of the South African Lowveld: Discourse, Accusations and Subjective Reality," *Journal of the Royal Anthropological Institute* 11, no. 2 (2015): 191–210.

6. Mark Auslander, "Open the Wombs! The Symbolic Politics of Ngoni Witchfinding," in *Modernity and Its Malcontents: Ritual and Power in Postcolonial Africa*, ed. Jean Comaroff and John L. Comaroff (Chicago: University of Chicago Press), 167–192.

7. Niehaus, Mohlale, and Shokane, *Witchcraft, Power and Politics*, 154.

208 NOTES TO PAGES 99–121

8. Jonathan Metzl, *Dying of Whiteness: How Racial Resentment Is Killing America's Heartland* (New York: Basic Books, 2019); Steve Biko, *I Write What I Like: Selected Writings* (Chicago: University of Chicago Press, 1978).

9. Hugo ka Canham, *Riotous Deathscapes* (Durham, NC: Duke University Press, 2023); vangile gantsho, *red cotton* (Tshwane, South Africa: impepho press, 2018); Casey Golomski, *Funeral Culture: AIDS, Work and Cultural Change in an African Kingdom* (Bloomington: Indiana University Press, 2018); Niehaus, Mohlale, and Shokane, *Witchcraft, Power and Politics*.

10. William C. Olsen and Walter E. A. van Beek, eds., *Evil in Africa: Encounters with the Everyday* (Bloomington: Indiana University Press, 2015), 12–13.

11. This comparison has been made before in thinking about American cultures of Karens, racism, and witches: Regina Jackson and Saira Rao, *White Women: Everything You Already Know about Your Own Racism and How to Do Better* (New York: Penguin, 2020), 139–140; Ligaya Mishan, "The March of the Karens," *New York Times Magazine*, August 12, 2021.

JOKERS

1. Isak Niehaus, "Coins for Blood, and Blood for Coins: From Sacrifice to Ritual Murder in the South African Lowveld, 1930–2000," *Etnofoor* 13, no. 2 (2000): 31–54.

2. "Bungalile utshuala (Drinking is not good for me)," track 6 on Hugh Tracey, *Dances and Songs for Running and Walking by the Swazi People of Swaziland*, International Library of African Music ILAMTR073, 1958, digital.

3. Toyin Owoseje, "Charlize Theron Faces Backlash after Saying Afrikaans, Her Mother Tongue, Is Dying Out," CNN, November 18, 2022, https://www.cnn.com/2022/11/18/enter tainment/charlize-theron-afrikaans-backlash-south-africa-intl-scli/index.html.

4. Kees de Bot and Sinfree Makoni, eds., *Language and Aging in Multilingual Contexts* (Clevedon, UK: Multilingual Matters, 2005).

5. Ta-Nehisi Coates, "The Case for Reparations," *Atlantic*, June 15, 2014. See also William Darity and A. Kirsten Mullen, *From Here to Equality: Reparations for Black Americans in the Twenty-First Century* (Chapel Hill: University of North Carolina Press, 2020).

6. Janet McIntosh, *Unsettled: Denial and Belonging among White Kenyans* (Durham, NC: Duke University Press, 2016); Scott Burnett, *White Belongings: Race, Land, and Property in Post-Apartheid South Africa* (Lanham, MD: Lexington Books, 2022).

7. Lauren Berlant and Sian Ngai, "Comedy Has Issues: An Introduction," *Critical Inquiry* 43, no. 2 (2017): 233–249.

8. Grace Musila, "Laughing at the Rainbow's Cracks? Blackness, Whiteness and the Ambivalence of South African Stand-Up Comedy," in *Civic Agency in Africa: Arts of Resistance in the 21st Century*, ed. Ebenezer Obadare and W. Willems (Suffolk, UK: James Currey, 2014), 147–166.

9. See Casey Golomski, "Greying Mutuality: Race and Joking Relations in a South African Nursing Home," *Africa* 90, no. 2 (2020): 273–292.

YVONNE

1. Luise White, *Fighting and Writing: The Rhodesian Army at War and Postwar* (Durham, NC: Duke University Press, 2022).

2. *All Quiet on the Western Front*, dir. Edward Berger (Berlin: Amusement Park Film GmbH, 2022).

3. Matthias Häussler, *The Herero Genocide: War, Emotion, and Extreme Violence in Colonial Namibia*, trans. Elizabeth Janik (New York: Berghahn Books, 2021).

4. Philip Oltermann, "German Critics Pan Oscar-Nominated All Quiet on the Western Front," *Guardian*, January 27, 2023.

5. Kate Law, "Mostly We Are White and Alone: Identity, Anxiety and the Past in Some White Zimbabwean Memoirs," *Journal of Historical Sociology* 29, no. 3 (2016): 297–318.

6. George Bishi, "Immigration and Settlement of 'Undesirable' Whites in Southern Rhodesia, c. 1940s–1960s," in *Rethinking White Societies in Southern Africa, 1930s–1990s*, ed. Duncan

NOTES TO PAGES 131–141

Money and Danelle van Zyl-Hermann (London: Routledge, 2020), 59–77; Alfred Tembo and Jochen Lingelbach, "The Forgotten History of Migration to Africa," *Africa Is a Country*, January 25, 2021.

GOD

1. Ivan Fallon, "My Deathbed Conversation with FW de Klerk, the Leader Who Killed Apartheid," *Sunday Times*, November 14, 2021, https://www.thetimes.co.uk/article/my-deathbed-conversation-with-fw-de-klerk-the-leader-who-killed-apartheid-cqmjvo9dt.

2. Christi van der Westhuizen, "FW de Klerk: The Last Apartheid President Was Driven by Pragmatism, Not Idealism," *The Conversation*, November 11, 2021, https://theconversation.com/fw-de-klerk-the-last-apartheid-president-was-driven-by-pragmatism-not-idealism-164026.

3. Ilana van Wyk, *The Universal Church of the Kingdom of God in South Africa: A Church of Strangers* (Cambridge: Cambridge University Press, 2014).

4. See Antjie Krog's poem "Land" in her collection *Down to My Last Skin* (Johannesburg: Random House, 2000).

MAMA ZULU

1. Jonathan Graff-Radford, "Sundowning: Late-Day Confusion," Expert Answers, Mayo Clinic, May 27, 2022.

2. Crain Soudien, "Constituting the Class: An Analysis of the Process of 'Integration' in South African Schools," in *Changing Class: Education and Social Change in Post-Apartheid South Africa*, ed. Linda Chisholm (Pretoria: HSRC Press, 2004), 89–114; Krisztina Z. Tihanyi and Stephanos F. du Toit, "Reconciliation through Integration? An Examination of South Africa's Reconciliation Process in Racially Integrating High Schools," *Conflict Resolution Quarterly* 23, no. 1 (2005): 25–41; Mary Pattillo, "The Problem of Integration," in *The Dream Revisited: Contemporary Debates about Housing, Segregation, and Opportunity*, ed. Ingrid Ellen and Justin Steil (New York: Columbia University Press, 2019), 29–32.

3. Steve Biko, *I Write What I Like: Selected Writings* (Chicago: University of Chicago Press, 1978); Tiffany Lethabo King, Jenell Navaro, and Andrew Smith, eds., *Otherwise Worlds: Against Settler Colonialism and Anti-Blackness* (Durham, NC: Duke University Press, 2020).

4. Charl Blignaut, "'Die Hand Aan Die Wieg Regeer Die Land [The Hand That Rocks the Cradle Rules the Land]': Exploring the Agency and Identity of Women in the Ossewa-Brandwag, 1939–1954," *South African Historical Journal* 67, no. 1 (2015): 47–63; Marijke du Toit, "Women, Welfare and the Nurturing of Afrikaner Nationalism: A Social History of the Afrikaanse Christelike Vroue Vereniging, c. 1870–1939" (PhD diss., University of Cape Town, 1996).

5. Renugan Raidoo, "Clearing Space: Postapartheid Liberalism and the Evolution of Spatial Segregation in Johannesburg's New Urban Enclaves" (PhD diss., Harvard University, 2022).

6. Keeanga-Yamahtta Taylor, *Race for Profit: How Banks and the Real Estate Industry Undermined Black Homeownership* (Chapel Hill: University of North Carolina Press, 2019).

7. Phehello Mofokeng, "Andizi! Black Tax Is a Flawed Social Construct," in *Black Tax: Burden or Ubuntu?*, ed. Niq Mhlongo (Johannesburg: Jonathan Ball, 2019), 114.

8. Sukoluhle Nyathi, "The Burden of Black Tax Can Only Be Alleviated by Generational Wealth," in Mhlongo, *Black Tax*, 246–247.

9. Cati Coe, *Changes in Care: Aging, Migration and Social Change in West Africa* (New Brunswick, NJ: Rutgers University Press, 2019).

10. See Guy Harling et al., "Impairment in Activities of Daily Living, Care Receipt, and Unmet Needs in a Middle-Aged and Older Rural South African Population: Findings from the HAALSI Study," *Journal of Aging and Health* 32, nos. 5–6 (2020): 296–307; Ruimallo Herl et al., "Pension Exposure and Health: Evidence from a Longitudinal Study in South Africa," *Journal of Ageing and Economics* 23 (2022): 10411; and HAALSI: Health and Aging in Africa: A Longitudinal Study of an INDEPTH Community in South Africa, "Publications," Harvard University, accessed January 17, 2024, https://haalsi.org/publications.

11. Shireen Ally and Arianna Lissoni, eds., *New Histories of South Africa's Apartheid-Era Bantustans* (New York: Routledge, 2017); Shireen Ally, "Peaceful Memories: Remembering and Forgetting Political Violence in KaNgwane, South Africa," *Africa* 81, no. 3 (2011): 351–372; LeRoy Vail, ed., *The Creation of Tribalism in Southern Africa* (Berkeley: University of California Press, 1991).

12. See Elma Romy van Jaarsveld, "Water Supply and Quality of Life in Rural Settlements" (master's thesis, University of Pretoria, 2000), 37.

13. See "The Watchman's Blues," in Oswald Mbuyiseni Mtshali's collection *Song of the Cowhide Drum* (New York: Third Press, 1972), 51.

14. Ally, "Peaceful Memories," 356.

15. See Public Health and Social Development Sectoral Bargaining Council [South Africa], *Resolution 1 of 2022: Agreement on the Provision of Uniform for Nurses in the Public Health and Social Development Sector*, 1–6, https://www.phsdsbc.org.za/wp-content/uploads/2022/05 /Agreement-of-the-Provision-of-Uniform-for-Nurses-1.pdf.

16. On the park wildfires that killed over twenty Swati women grasscutters in 2001, see Jacob Dlamini, *Safari Nation: A Social History of the Kruger National Park* (Auckland Park, Johannesburg: Jacana, 2020), 229.

SECURITY

1. Aryn Baker, "This Photo Galvanized the World against Apartheid: Here's the Story behind It," *Time LightBox*, June 5, 2016, https://time.com/4365138/soweto-anniversary -photograph/.

2. "Keep It in the Family, Begs Hector Pieterson's Sister," *Mail and Guardian*, March 22, 2013, https://mg.co.za/article/2013-03-22-00-keep-it-in-the-family-begs-hector-pietersons-sister/.

3. Joshua P. Murphy et al., "Community Health Worker Models in South Africa: A Qualitative Study on Policy Implementation of the 2018/19 Revised Framework," *Healthy Policy and Planning* 36, no. 4 (May 2021): 384–396.

4. Jessica Ruthven, "Suffering Grannies," in *Connected Lives: Families, Households, Health and Care in Contemporary South Africa*, ed. Nolwazi Mkhwanazi and Lenore Manderson (Cape Town: Human Sciences Research Council, 2020), 181.

5. Again, the euphemism for a low CD4 white blood cell count, and HIV/AIDS complications in general.

6. Tiffany Lethabo King, Jenell Navaro, and Andrew Smith, eds., *Otherwise Worlds: Against Settler Colonialism and Anti-Blackness* (Durham, NC: Duke University Press, 2020).

7. Shaka McGlotten, "Always towards a Black Queer Anthropology," *Transforming Anthropology* 20, no. 1 (2012): 3–4.

8. Christine Obbo, "'But We Know It All!' African Perspectives on Anthropological Knowledge," in *African Anthropologies*, ed. Mwenda Ntarangwi, David Mills, and Mustafa Babiker (Dakar: CODESRIA, 2006), 154.

NOELINE

1. See Dean McCleland, "Port Elizabeth of Yore: From Sundridge to Sharley Cribb," *The Casual Observer*, July 15, 2019, http://thecasualobserver.co.za/port-elizabeth-of-yore-from -sundridge-to-the-sharley-cribb/; Vanessa Noble, "Doctors Divided: Gender, Race and Class Anomalies in the Production of Black Medical Doctors in Apartheid South Africa, 1948–1994" (PhD diss., University of Michigan, 2005), 50.

2. Christo Brand, with Barbara Jones, *Mandela: My Prisoner, My Friend* (London: John Blake, 2014), 31.

3. Robben Island Museum and World Heritage, "Historical Background to the *Suzan Kruger* Ferry," South African Heritage Resources Agency, accessed March 23, 2023, https:// tinyurl.com/SAHRAsuzankruger.

4. See Robben Island Museum, "Introduction," in *Robben Island World Heritage Site Integrated Conservation Management Plan (2013–2018)* (Cape Town: Robben Island World Heritage Site, 2013).

NOTES TO PAGES 167–180

5. Nelson Mandela and Mandla Langa, *Dare Not Linger: The Presidential Years* (New York: Farrar, Straus and Giroux, 2017), 210. Mandela also argued, "The black warders, also victims of the violence driving the apartheid policy, which had turned them into instruments of their own oppression, were a mostly more benighted version of their paler brethren" (210).

6. Andrew Thompson, "'Restoring Hope Where All Hope Was Lost': Nelson Mandela, the ICRC and the Protection of Political Detainees in Apartheid South Africa," *International Review of the Red Cross* 98, no. 903 (2016): 799–829. Georg Hoffmann was the first ICRC inspector to see Robben Island and meet the prisoners in August 1964. Likely fearing the prevention of future visits there, Hoffmann's report was subdued, and the apartheid state cherry-picked parts of it to publish in the South African press in 1966 to misrepresent the prison's actual conditions. Godfrey Senn's later inspection on April 5–10, 1967, included photographs and recorded interviews with Mandela. While sympathetic toward the cause, "he became, as Mandela—with typical restraint—observed, acclimatized to the very racism of which he was a critic" (Thompson, "'Restoring Hope,'" 805).

7. Brand, *Mandela*, 39.

8. Brand, *Mandela*, 125–126.

9. Fran Lisa Buntman, *Robben Island and Prisoner Resistance to Apartheid* (Cambridge: Cambridge University Press, 2003), 197–202.

10. Brand, *Mandela*, 61.

11. Nelson Mandela, "The Ward," Belgravia Gallery, accessed January 24, 2024, https://belgraviagallery.com/artist/nelson-mandela/the-ward/.

12. Mandela, "Ward."

13. Katy Kelleher, "Chartreuse, the Color of Elixirs, Flappers, and Alternate Realities," *Paris Review*, December 17, 2018.

14. Eric Allen Hall, "'I Guess I'm Becoming More and More Militant': Arthur Ashe and the Black Freedom Movement, 1961–1968," *Journal of African American History* 96, no. 4 (2011): 474–502; Marion Keim and Lyndon Bouah, "Sport and Recreation on Robben Island," *International Journal of the History of Sport* 30, no. 16 (2013): 1962–1975.

15. Brand, *Mandela*, 61. Brand wrote that Mandela was seen by a (male) medical officer every day who acted on a government doctor's orders. The doctor came once a week from the mainland, along with periodic visits by a dentist and a fortnightly visit by a psychiatrist. Also, "like all prisoners his age, Mandela has annual medical checkups on the mainland" (61) and met with an eye doctor for quarry-related injuries and an otolaryngologist. These mainland trips were clandestine as wardens feared it was an opportunity for prisoners to escape. While Mandela met with these doctors, Brand stood outside the consult room with a 9mm handgun. His colleagues carried machine guns. "Luckily, Mandela never really seemed to get sick at this time. He would perhaps have cough medicine occasionally, but that was all" (57).

16. Sean Field, "'What Can I Do When the Interviewee Cries?' Oral History Strategies for Containment and Regeneration," in *Oral History in a Wounded Country: Interactive Interviewing in South Africa*, ed. Phillipe Denis and Radikobo Ntsimane (Scottsville: University of KwaZulu-Natal Press, 2008), 144–168.

17. Pumla Gobodo-Madikizela, *A Human Being Died That Night: A South African Woman Confronts the Legacy of Apartheid* (Boston: Mariner, 2003), 86.

THE CIRCLE

1. Ervin Goffman, *Frame Analysis: An Essay on the Organization of Experience* (London: Harper and Row, 1974).

2. Marie Jorritsma, *Sonic Spaces of the Karoo: The Sacred Music of a South African Coloured Community* (Philadelphia: Temple University Press, 2011); Hugo ka Canham, *Riotous Deathscapes* (Durham, NC: Duke University Press, 2023).

3. Zakes Mda, *The Madonna of Excelsior* (New York: Picador, 2002).

4. Justine van der Leun, "The Odd Couple: Why an Apartheid Activist Joined Forces with a Murderer," *Guardian*, June 6, 2015.

5. Pumla Gobodo-Madikizela, *A Human Being Died That Night: A South African Woman Confronts the Legacy of Apartheid* (Boston: Mariner, 2003).

6. Truth and Reconciliation Commission of South Africa, *Final Report*, vol. 2 (Pretoria: Department of Justice, 1998).

7. Van der Leun, "Odd Couple."

8. Ali Mphaki, "Daughter of Victim Forgives De Kock," *IOL*, February 13, 2012.

9. Tim Butcher, "Witch Doctors 'Cleanse' Vlakplaas," *Telegraph*, December 17, 2001.

10. "State Gets Vlakplaas Back after 20 Years," News24, July 20, 2014, https://www.news24.com/news24/state-gets-vlakplaas-back-after-20-years-20150429.

CONFESSIONS

1. Michael Jackson, *Minima Ethnographica: Intersubjectivity and the Anthropological Project* (Chicago: University of Chicago Press, 1998); Michael Jackson, *Critique of Identity Thinking* (New York: Berghahn Books, 2019).

2. James H. Cone, *A Black Theology of Liberation* (Maryknoll, NY: Orbis Books, 1986), 73; Darryl Scriven, "Blue on Black Violence: Freddie Gray, Baltimore, South Africa, and the Question of Africana Christian Theology," *Journal of Pan African Studies* 8, no. 3 (2015): 119–126; M. Shawn Copeland, "The Grace of James Hal Cone," *CLR James Review* 25, nos. 1–2 (2019): 249–259; Sandisele L. Xhinti, "Revisiting Black Theology of Liberation in South Africa: Through 'New Voices' of Women Black Theologians," *Hervormde Teologiese Studies* 77, no. 3 (2021): e1–e9.

3. Roland Hill, "Black Grace—Part 2," *Spectrum Magazine*, February 25, 2021.

4. Hill, "Black Grace."

5. Dana Freibach-Heifetz, *Secular Grace* (Leiden: Brill, 2017); Kai Wiegandt, "The Creature-Feeling as Secular Grace: On the Religious in J.M. Coetzee's Fiction," *Literature and Theology* 32, no. 1 (2018): 69–86; Samuel Huard, "The Otherwise and Grace: Exploring Theopolitical Connections," *Studies in Religion/Sciences Religieuses* (December 9, 2023), doi: 10.1177/00084298231212200.

6. Sara Ahmed, "Declarations of Whiteness: The Non-Performativity of Anti-Racism," *borderlands* 3, no. 2 (2004).

7. William Darity and A. Kirsten Mullen, *From Here to Equality: Reparations for Black Americans in the Twenty-First Century* (Chapel Hill: University of North Carolina Press, 2020); Melanie Judge and Dee Smythe, eds., *Unsettling Apologies: Critical Writings on Apology from South Africa* (Bristol, UK: Bristol University Press, 2022).

8. Everett L. Worthington Jr. and Nathaniel G. Wade, eds., *Handbook of Forgiveness*, 2nd ed. (New York: Routledge, 2020); Arzoo Osanloo, *Forgiveness Work: Mercy, Law and Victims' Rights in Iran* (Princeton, NJ: Princeton University Press, 2020); Judge and Smythe, *Unsettling Apologies*.

9. Sisonke Msimang, "Rescuing Mandela from Sainthood," *Africa Is a Country*, April 27, 2019.

10. Marvin E. Wickware Jr., "For the Love of (Black) Christ: Embracing James Cone's Affective Critique of White Fragility, *Toronto Journal of Theology* 33, no. 1 (2017): 103.

11. Wickware, "For the Love of (Black) Christ," 103.

12. Melissa Steyn, *Whiteness Just Isn't What It Used to Be: White Identity in a Changing South Africa* (Albany: State University of New York Press, 2001); Christi van der Westhuizen, *Sitting Pretty: White Afrikaans Women in Postapartheid South Africa* (Scottsville: University of KwaZulu-Natal Press, 2017); Barnor Hesse, "Black Populism," *Southern Atlantic Quarterly* 121, no. 3 (2022): 561–592.

13. Sarah Lamb, "Permanent Personhood or Meaningful Decline? Toward a Critical Anthropology of Successful Aging," *Journal of Aging Studies* 29 (2014): 41–52; Sarah Lamb, ed., *Successful Aging as a Contemporary Obsession: Global Perspectives* (New Brunswick, NJ: Rutgers University Press, 2017).

14. Simone de Beauvoir, *The Coming of Age*, trans. Patrick O'Brian (New York: W. W. Norton, [1970] 1996); Gail Weiss, "The Myth of Woman Meets the Myth of Old Age: An Alienating

NOTES TO PAGES 189–191

Encounter with the Aging Female Body," in *Simone de Beauvoir's Philosophy of Age: Gender, Ethics, and Time*, ed. Silvia Stoller (Boston: De Gruyter, 2014), 47–64; Silke van Dyk and Thomas Küpper, eds., "Theorizing Age—Postcolonial Perspectives in Aging Studies," special issue, *Journal of Aging Studies* 39 (2016); Sweta Rajan-Rankin, "Race, Embodiment and Later Life: Re-Animating Aging Bodies of Color," *Journal of Aging Studies* 45 (2018): 32–38.

15. On the radical potential of dis-identification, or un-becoming, as a racial, gendered, and anti-essentializing political act, see Chantal Mouffe, "Feminism, Citizenship, and Radical Democratic Politics," in *Chantal Mouffe: Hegemony, Radical Democracy, and the Political*, ed. James Martin (London: Routledge, [1992] 2013), 132–145; Jóse Esteban Muñoz, *Disidentifications: Queers of Color and the Performance of Politics* (Minneapolis: University of Minnesota Press, 1999); Christine Clark and James O'Donnell, eds., *Becoming and Unbecoming White: Owning and Disowning a Racial Identity* (Westport, CT: Bergin & Garvey, 1999); Joaõ H. Costa Vargas, "Black Radical Becoming: The Politics of Identification in Permanent Transformation," *Critical Sociology* 32, nos. 2–3 (2006): 475–500; Danai S. Mupotsa, "Becoming Girl-Woman-Bride," *Girlhood Studies* 8, no. 3 (2015): 73–87; João Biehl and Peter Locke, eds., *Unfinished: The Anthropology of Becoming* (Durham, NC: Duke University Press, 2017); Hans Asenbaum, "The Politics of Becoming: Disidentification as Radical Democratic Practice," *European Journal of Social Theory* 24, no. 1 (2020): 86–104; "Hesse, "Black Populism."

16. Msimang, "Rescuing Mandela."

17. Msimang, "Rescuing Mandela."

18. M. Wolff, personal communication, August 7, 2023. Thank you for the wisdom, M., and for the final endnote. See also Julian Pitt-Rivers, "The Place of Grace in Anthropology," *Hau* 1, no. 1 (2011 [1992]): 423–450; Omri Elisha, "Moral Ambitions of Grace: The Paradox of Compassion and Accountability in Evangelical Faith-Based Activism," *Cultural Anthropology* 23, no. 1 (2008): 154–189; Vincent Lloyd, *The Problem of Grace: Reconfiguring Political Theology* (Stanford, CA: Stanford University Press, 2011); Michael Edwards and Méadhbh McIvor, eds., "'Always Something Extra': Ethnographies of Grace," special issue, *Cambridge Journal of Anthropology* 40, no. 1 (2022); Neena Mahadev, *Karma and Grace: Religious Difference in Millennial Sri Lanka* (New York: Columbia University Press, 2023).

Index

acceptance, 4, 74, 81, 121, 154, 182, 185–192; unequal racial reckoning, 188–189
activities of daily living, 85
admissions policies, 125, 136, 150, 156, 164, 175
Affordable Care Act (Obamacare), 7, 9, 22
African National Congress (ANC), 47–48, 81, 95, 190
afterlife, 20, 130, 133–134, 192; *lahlabantu* (rite after a death), 134
age as honorable, 3–4, 75, 81, 137, 144, 189
age groups, terminology for, 3
ageism, 4, 9, 13, 64, 114, 162, 184, 189; nonhuman stereotypes, 16
Age of Iron (Coetzee), 15
Agincourt community district (South Africa), 141
aging: "gracefully," 17, 189; "successfully," 189; as universal, 17. *See also* gerotranscendence theories
aging in place, 10, 59, 104; as security issue, 182
"Agric Alert," 119
AIDS pandemic, 93, 162. *See also* HIV, living with
Airbnb cottages ("granny flats"), 38
All Quiet on the Western Front (Remarque), 120
Alzheimer's and dementia, x, 21, 47, 94, 99–100, 109, 132, 141, 157–158, 188–189, 192; films about, 78–79; and haunting, 109; "sundowning," 137; violence toward old people with, 161–162
"Amazing Grace," 132
ancestors, 19–20, 49, 114, 157, 173, 177–178, 181; and afterlife, 134, 147; chiefs and kings as, 134; and healers, 100, 144. *See also* ghosts
Andrea Boccelli Live in Central Park, 128

Anglican Church, 26, 55, 56
apartheid, vii–viii, 1; anti-apartheid struggle, 47–48, 96–97, 152–153; development and expansion of, 11–12; educational policies, 152–153, 179; gambling banned under, 42; "homelands," 12, 96, 101–103, 142–143, 202n17; marriage laws, 55; "native reserves" policies, 11–12; official end of in 1994, viii, 8, 12, 58, 81; supposed ending of, 8, 161; "tribal authorities," 142; Vlakplaas, 180–182
Ashe, Arthur, 169
Autshumo (Khoi leader), 167

baby boomers, United States, 10, 14, 49, 83
Badenhorst, Piet, 168
Baldwin, James, 167
Barnard, Christian, 124
Bechuanaland, 121. *See also* Botswana
belonging, 52, 69, 101, 113–114, 136, 138, 187
Benoni (Johannesburg suburb), 53, 56–57
Berlant, Lauren, 114
Berlin Conference of 1884–1885, 120
Biden, Joe, 49
Big Love (HBO series), 157
Bill of Rights (South Africa), 27
Bismarck, Otto von, 119–120
"black," as term, xi
Black Authorities Act (1962), 142
"Black Grace," 185
black liberation theologians, 185, 187
black people: as domestic workers, 45, 141; evictions of, 27, 31, 87, 101, 142; family farms, 2; joking, 113–114; middle-class, 139–141; political perspectives, 47, 81, 114. *See also* African National Congress (ANC); caregivers

215

Black Tax: Burden or Ubuntu? (Mhlongo), 77, 140–141
Blignaut, Charl, 139
Bonthuys, Cecilia, 55
borders, 89, 117, 142–143; between this world and the next, 20
Botswana, 121. *See also* Bechuanaland
Brand, Christo, 168, 211n15
Bremer, Karl, 164
Brooks, Garth, 82–83
Buntman, Fran Lisa, 168
burdens, 77, 140–141, 154, 162, 189
Burkhard, Simon, 168

Cape Party, 13
Cape Town, 89, 112, 121, 166–167, 170
capit(abl)ism, 63
caregivers: education for, 38, 94–96; night shifts, 35, 106–107; racism faced by, 78–79, 105, 126–127, 188; wages, 83–84, 160; working-class women and women of color as, viii, 16–17, 78, 141, 162. *See also* nurses
caregiving: by family, 77, 104, 125, 140–141, 148–151, 155, 174; and power, 131; shaped by racism, 78–79
Carnegie Corporation, 10
"Case for Reparations, The" (Coates), 113
character, 3, 105, 185
charities, 10, 42–43, 139, 154
circle of life, 89, 174, 176–177
Civil Union Act (2006), 55
Coates, Ta-Nehisi, 113
Coetzee, J. M., 15, 141
colonialism, 14, 25, 47, 54, 64, 109, 119, 121, 167, 178; and corruption discourses, 81; critiques of, 63–64
colorblind discourse, 17, 106, 126, 170
coloured, as racial category, 200n4
Commonwealth of Nations, 55
complaining, 32, 36, 50–51, 73, 125–128, 162
Comrades (youth group), 96–101, 146
confessions, 4, 97, 99, 100, 133, 186–187
conspiracies, 14, 106
conversational narrative, ix–x
Correctional Services, 48, 163, 165, 168
corruption discourses, 41–42, 48, 81–82, 94, 98, 105, 130, 193
COVID-19, 16, 28–31, 38, 95, 156; race differences in hospital admissions, 31; in United States, 83
Crapanzano, Vincent, 14–15
Cribb, Sharley, 164
"crisis committees," 95. *See also* Comrades (youth group)
critical diversity studies, 63

Davey, Bill, 53–54
Day Apartheid Died, The (photo), 152–153
daytime activity centers for older adults, 98, 155
death, 33, 176–182; and circle of life, 89, 174, 176–177; life carries on, 33, 34, 130; *lahlabantu* (rite after a death), 134; royalty not mourned, 15
"deathbed confessions," 100, 176–179
"death panels," 7
DeBeers, 9
dehumanization of older adults, 96–99. *See also* "witches" and witchfinders
de Klerk, F. W., 131, 190
de Kock, Eugene, 180–181
Deokoran, Babita, 81–82
Department of Social Development, 154
diminutives, used for older adults, 36–37, 110
dis-identification, 17, 133, 185, 189–190, 213n15
dis-integration, 17, 185, 188–190
diversity training workshop, 62–66, 68–69. *See also* integration
domestic workers, 15–16, 45, 57–58, 89, 141
Donham, Carolyn Bryant, 13
Dream House, The (Higginson), 15–16, 141
Dutch East India Company, 112
Dutch Reformed Church, 178
du Toit, Andries, 69

Economic Freedom Fighters (EFF), 28, 81, 114
education, 94–95; apartheid policies, 179; "separate-but-equal" medical education, 164
elder abuse, 78
Elder Justice Act, 7
electrification, 28, 41, 101–102
elephants, 42, 117, 129; and circle of life, 89
Elizabeth II, 14
"Elsewhere," 4, 5, 95, 120, 155. *See also* "Otherwise" worlds
emakosi (spirits of chiefs and kings), 134–135
emergency rooms, 16, 29, 163; off-loaded patients, 107
empathy, 185, 190
empowerment, 14, 27, 130, 187–189
entertainment, 71, 74, 77–78, 133
equality, 45–46, 105, 113–114, 182; in Bill of Rights, 25
Equality Court, 13
erasure, viii
Eskom, 42
eSwatini, Kingdom of, 142–143; as absolute monarchy, 35, 159
evictions of black people, 27, 31, 87, 101, 142

INDEX   217

"failures": "poor" people stereotypes in
    United States, 146; seen as witches, 97, 100
family, caregiving by, 140–141, 148–151, 155
Finn, Reygan, 60
forest estates (timber plantations), 107, 117,
    119, 181
forgiveness, 14, 105, 171, 181, 187
Fouche, J. J., 166
Fourie, Marié Adriaana, 55
Freud, Sigmund, x
"F-CKWHITEPEOPLE" print (Hutton),
    12–13
"F-ck your Racist Grandma" slogan, 2–3,
    12–13
funding for old age homes, 21–24, 138–140;
    after apartheid, 45–46; charity donations,
    42–43, 154, 156; from churches, 46; items
    for sale, 7, 44–45

gambling, regulated, 42
Gawande, Atul, 192
"gay voice," 53
GEMS (Government Employees Medical
    Scheme), 9
gender, xi, 17, 55, 74, 90, 91, 138, 159, 186;
    divide between nursing and corrections,
    170; gendered pronouns in black African
    languages, 130–131. See also dis-identifica-
    tion; sexism
generations, viii, 2–4, 9, 10, 17, 57, 89, 96,
    120–121, 191; contrasts between, 58,
    98–99, 104, 114, 117, 143, 188; generational
    curses, 100, 162; multigenerational
    households, 22, 99, 140. See also baby
    boomers; Comrades (youth group);
    Millennials
Genesis, 53
gerotranscendence theories, x, 191–192
Ghana, 141
ghosts, viii, 2, 4–5, 81, 145, 173; emakosi
    (spirits of chiefs and kings), 134–135; imali
    letipoko (ghosts' money), 109; and joking,
    114; next generation of, 4; "old ways of
    thinking" as, 2; of rainbow image, 27. See
    also ancestors
Gobodo-Madikizela, Pumla, 173, 180
God, 129–136; as collective power, 131; and
    gender, 130–131; and judgment, 131–133; as
    Mkulunkulu (the Great One), 131, 146.
    See also religion
Goffman, Erving, 176
"gogo," as term for grandmother, 3, 137
Gqola, Pumla, 66
grace, viii, x–xi, 184–192, 195; as acceptance,
    185–188; in action, 191; "Black Grace," 185;
    "divine grace," 185; "secular grace," 186

Grace (old age home): black residents in, 35,
    42, 95, 137–138, 141–142; bus plan, 25, 71, 85;
    Care Buddies program, 71, 74, 80, 94, 99,
    104, 125; graves on site of, 24, 27, 48–49,
    69–70, 86, 109, 135–136, 142; kitchen staff,
    41; night shifts, 106; residents' conditions
    discussed, 36–38; said to be like a family,
    vii, 5, 26, 32, 184, 186
grants. See older person grants
graves, disputes over, 24, 27, 48–49, 68–70,
    86, 87, 109, 134–136
"great wars" (World Wars I and II), 119–121

HAALSI ("Health and Aging in Africa:
    A Longitudinal Study of an INDEPTH
    Community in South Africa"), 141
Hani, Chris, 47–48
haunting, vii–viii, 4, 20, 22, 53, 109, 115,
    145, 191
healers. See sangoma, inyanga, dingaka
    (healers)
Health and Welfare Sector Education and
    Training Authority, 95
hearing aids, 49, 62, 112
heartsores, 38, 47, 99, 151, 183
Heritage Month, 86, 146
Higginson, Craig, 15–16, 141
Hill, Roland, 185
histoplasmosis, 28–29
HIV, living with, 95, 158; CD4 blood count,
    93, 207n2; screenings, 93; "soldiers," as
    euphemism for white blood cells, 93, 95.
    See also AIDS pandemic
Hoffman, Georg, 211n6
"homelands," 12, 96; Gazankulu, 96,
    101–103, 202n17; KaNgwane, 35, 142–143.
    See also townships
homelessness, 27
hospice, 23, 25, 30, 32, 201n11; "comfort
    measures only," 131
hospitals, public, 31, 35, 38–39. See also
    Themba (public hospital)
housing: under apartheid, 27; prices, 24–25;
    Reconstruction and Development Pro-
    gramme (RDP), 27–28; United States,
    60. See also real estate practices
Human Being Died That Night, A (Gobodo-
    Madikizela), 180
Hutton, Dean, 13
Hynes, Samuel, 119

Imago dei theology, 74, 129, 192
Immorality Act of 1950, 55, 179
independence, sense of, 39, 85, 139
independent living options for older adults,
    24, 49, 109, 136, 139–140, 156

218   INDEX

Indigenous Knowledge Secretariat, 181
Institute for Poverty, Land, and Agrarian
   Studies, 69
institutions, 167, 170; institutionalism, 138;
   for children, 121
integration, 41–42, 58; criticisms of, 138; in
   old-age homes, 21, 24, 26; United States,
   41. *See also* diversity training workshop
interdependence, viii–ix
International Committee of the Red Cross
   (ICRC), 167–168, 211n6
intersex people, 72–74, 80
intersubjective potential, 185
intimacy, sacred, 89
isolation, 29, 91, 95, 123, 141, 156, 186; political use of, 190

Jackson, Samuel L., 78–79
Jehovah's Witnesses, 62, 84, 146
joking, 108–115, 146, 157; and religion,
   129–130; about land theft, 112–114; alternative place and time created by, 114; fear
   masquerading as laughter, 113; in multiple
   languages, 111–112; "new normative constraints," 114

Kabasa gang, 146
ka Canham, Hugo, 28
Karade, Olatiwa, 3
Khan, Jamil, 60
Khisimus (Christmas), 45–46
Khoza, Marcia, 180–181
khulu, as term for old, 74
Kona, Bongani, 89
Krog, Antjie, 136
Kruger, Jimmy, 166
Kruger, Paul, 87, 109; *imali lePawula* (Paul's
   money), 109
Kruger National Park, 30, 86–92, 97, 108–109,
   152; black people forcibly removed from, 87,
   142; Numbi border gate, 73; self-segregation
   in, 90; wildlife, 86–90

labaphansi (the dead), 144
lahlabantu (rite after a death), 134
Lamb, Sarah, 189
land claims, 160; and graves, 24, 68–69; by
   Mdluli clan, 142–143. *See also* graves,
   disputes over
Land Claims Court, 69
"land grab," 68–70
land reform policy initiatives, 69, 113–114
languages: Afrikaans, 25, 111; black African,
   and gendered pronouns, 130–131; Fanagalo, 111–112; Shangaan, 42, 153; siSwati,
   25, 35, 43, 73, 111, 134, 161, 204n10; Xhosa,
   35, 99; Zulu, 25, 35. *See also* joking

Last Days of Ptolemy Gray, The (film), 78–79
Le Brun, Charles, 63
Le Guin, Ursula K., ix
Lekazi (Nsikazi settlement), 142, 146
Lesbian and Gay Equality Project, 55
LGBTQ+ people, 51–61; "gay voice," 53;
   "knowing," 51–52, 58; and old age homes,
   51–60; open secrets, 51–52, 60. *See also*
   intersex people
LGBTQ Senior Housing, Inc., 60
life carries on, 33, 34
life expectancy, 3, 8, 13–14, 17, 26, 188
liminal zones, 7
loan sharks, 23
long-term care: and social work, 19–20;
   United States, 10, 20
love, 77, 173–174, 191; as acceptance, 187–188

mabhalane (secretary bird), 135
Machadodorp (Ntokozweni), 178–179
Madonna, 17
Madonna of Excelsior, The (Mda), 179
Mahushu (town), 73, 86
Makhubo, Mbuyisa, 152–153
Mali, Zoli, 26
Malopa, Grandpa (black community
   trustee), 48–49, 69, 109, 135, 160
Mandela, Nelson, 4, 33, 47, 58, 81, 97, 131,
   190, 211nn5–6; medical visits, 211n15; at
   Robben Island prison, 163, 167
Mandela, Winnie, 81
maps: Google Maps, 9, 42; white names on,
   ix, 1–2, 5, 64, 85, 166, 195
marriage: *kushada*, 145; *lobola* (bride-
   wealth), 145; reflections on, 30, 55–56, 61,
   77, 100, 123, 145–146, 157, 165–166
Marriage Act, 55
marriage laws, 55
Mashobane, Derek, 181
Mass General (Boston), 125
Matthew, Gospel of, 93
Mbombela (Nelspruit) (South Africa), 1–2,
   5, 38
Mda, Zakes, 179
Mdluli Authority, 142
Mdlulis (clan group), 142–143
medical aid and schemes, 8–9, 19, 29, 139
Medical Parole Advisory Board, 48
medical parole decisions, 48
medical records (Kardex), 35–36, 51, 94, 156
medication, 35–37, 107, 131, 161, 167, 169, 172,
   181, 185, 211n15
memories, 46–47, 87–89; of apartheid, 47,
   146, 152–153, 187; of care, 77, 154–155,
   167–172, 174; traumatic, 172–173; of youth,
   56, 73–75, 87–88, 101, 121–122, 142–143,
   165, 179

INDEX 219

Metzl, Jonathan, 14
Mhlongo, Niq, 77, 140–141
middle class, 14–15, 161, 188; black, 139–141
Millennials, 3, 56, 195
mining and mines, 9, 29, 56–57, 109, 112, 117, 123, 143, 146
mission statements, 6, 21
Mkhize, Linda, 60
Mofokeng, Phehello, 140–141
Mohale, Thabo, 181
Mohlale, Eliazaar "Jimmy," 97
Molefi, Antoinette, 152
morality, 20, 186, 188; immorality, 55, 162. *See also* Immorality Act of 1950
Morogoro Conference (Tanzania, 1969), 47
Moyo, Malik, 81
Mpumalanga (South Africa), 2, 8, 27
Msimang, Sisonke, 187, 190
Mugabe, Robert, 117, 120
music, 34–35, 44, 61, 82, 110, 128, 132
Musila, Grace, 114

Namibia, 93
Narayan, Kirin, ix
National Health Insurance (NHI) plan (South Africa), 8–9, 49, 69, 187
National Lottery, 42, 154
National Party, 11, 55, 167, 190
"native reserves" policies, 11–12
Nazis, former, 13
near-death experiences, 116–117
"Nessun Dorma" (Puccini), 128
Ngai, Sian, 114
Ngcukaitobi, Tembeka, 69
Niehaus, Isak, 96, 97, 99
Nkomo, Joshua, 117
nonracialism, 27
Nsikazi settlement, 142
nurses, 32–39, 71–84, 150, 154–155; prison nursing, 158; prison nursing, and gender, 170; ranks, 38; travel (agency) nurses, 83–84, 107; working conditions, 160–161. *See also* caregivers
Nyathi, Sukoluhle, 141
Nzima, Sam, 152–153

Obama, Barack, 7
old age, as category, 57
old age homes: for black older adults, 156; black professional views of, 140–141; black residents, 35, 42, 95, 104, 137–138, 141–142, 156, 161; as business, 24–25; consulting doctors, 38; fewer black residents in, 25, 35, 42, 139, 141; frail care and hospice options, 23–25, 32; funding for, 7, 42–46, 154, 156; integrated, 21, 24, 26; joking in,

108–112; and LGBTQ+ people, 51–60; move from upscale to subsidized care, 23–24; outings, 25, 71, 85, 86–92; "performances" by residents, 112, 137, 149; public-private differences, 139; security in, 9–10, 19, 32, 86, 153; turnover among workers, 83; visitors, 36, 43–44, 148–150; waiting lists, 125, 136, 150, 164, 175; waiting rooms, 6–7; whites-only, 10, 21. *See also* long-term care
older person grants, 21–23, 27, 36, 77; grant queues, 22–23; used by family, 150–151
"old ways of life/thinking," 2–4, 13–14. *See also* generations: contrasts between
"Otherwise" worlds, 4, 5, 96, 138, 155. *See also* "Elsewhere"

"participant framework," 176
peace, making, 81, 105. See *also* forgiveness; love
Philip, Prince, 14
Pieterson, Hector, 152–153
Plaatjieville, 69, 159
police, 94, 97, 98, 101; black double agents, 146; raids on farms, 181–182; shootings of protesters, 152–153
political parties, 28; unbanning of black, 12, 48
Pollsmoor Prison, 172, 190
power: collective, 131; and gender, 130–131; as godlike, 131
Powerball, 42
prison nursing, 158
Prohibition of Mixed Marriages Act of 1949, 55
protests, 41, 82, 152–153, 183; alleged "land grab," 68–70
Pryde, The, 60
Public Service Act (1994), 103
purgatory, 7

"queer," as term, 81

racism: caregiving shaped by, 78–79; and death penalty, 67; faced by care workers, 78, 105, 126–127, 188; "F-ck your Racist Grandma" slogan, 2–3, 12–13; and joking, 114; "Karens," 106, 190; and old age home admissions, 175; "race doesn't matter" linked to, 17; racist grandmas and grandpas, 2–4, 15; racists as "witches," 105–106
Raidoo, Renugan, 139
rainbow metaphor, 26–28
Rainbow Nation, 26, 58, 114
Ramaphosa, Cyril, 9
real estate practices, 24–25, 139–140

Reconstruction and Development Programme (RDP), 27–28
reflective narrative, ix–x
regrets and living in the past, 124–125
religion, 129; afterlife, 130, 133–135, 192; black liberation theologians, 185, 187; Christian narration of life journey, 146; churches, 15, 45–46, 55, 101, 132; "divine grace," 185; fire churches, 132; prosperity gospel, 132. *See also* God
Remarque, Erich Maria, 119–120
reparations, 113, 138
"Repealing the Job-Killing Health Care Law Act," 7
"replacement theories," 14
retirement, 9, 27, 30, 57, 61, 102, 158
Rhodes, Cecil, 47, 117
Rhodesia (Zimbabwe), 44, 47, 117–123; DC Office ("District Commissioner"), 119
Rhodesian Security Forces' Combined Operations program, 119
"RhodesMustFall" student movement, 47, 117
rites of passage, 7, 101
Rivonia Trial, 171
Robben Island prison, 33, 163, 166–173; black warders, 211n5; brutal conditions, 167; expanded to house more prisoners, 167; former prisoners as tour guides, 170; ICRC inspections, 167–168, 211n6; Mandela's depictions of, 169; political prisoners, 168, 171–172
Rob Ferreira (public hospital), 36, 38

Sachsenhausen concentration camp (Nazi Germany), 13
sangoma, inyanga, dingaka (healers), 100–101, 146–147, 153–154, 156; primary healthcare taught to, 158; training, 143–145
Schütz, Josef, 13
Second Anglo-Boer War, 139, 178
"secular grace," 186
Security (old age home), 104, 153–162; black residents in, 156; general wards rather than private rooms, 156–157; working conditions, 160–161
security, in old age homes, 9–10, 19, 32, 72, 86, 153
self-affirmation, 74–75
self-certitude, 4
Senn, Godfrey, 167–168, 211n6
separatism, 138
sexism, viii, 64–65, 78, 114, 184, 189
Shabangu, Portia, 180–181
Sharley Cribb Nursing College, 164
Shokane, Edith "Kally," 98

shopping, vii, 50–51, 70, 112
Simelane, Noks, 81
Sisulu, Walter, 172
"*Sizohamba naye!*" (We will walk with Him!) (hymn), 34–35
Skosana, Dineo, 24
Smit, Louis, 181
Smith, Ian, 119
Sobhuza I (Somhlolo), 113, 134–135
Sobhuza II (Paramount Chief and King of Swaziland, 135
social media, 2, 6, 106, 184, 195; *See also* X (formerly Twitter)
social work, 19–20, 26, 101, 162, 164
"soldiers," as euphemism for white blood cells, 93, 95
South Africa: agriculture, 2; Bill of Rights, 27; corruption discourses, 81–82, 94; death penalty abolished, 48, 66–67; grant queues, 22–23; Heritage Month, 86, 148; housing, 27–28; Immorality Act of 1950, 55, 179; land reform policy initiatives, 69, 113–114; leaves Commonwealth of Nations, 55; National Health Insurance (NHI) plan, 8; official languages, 26; older person grants, 21–23, 27; place name changes post-apartheid, 1, 27, 35, 38, 47, 177–178; protests, 41, 82, 152–153, 183; Public Service Act (1994), 103; Truth and Reconciliation Commission, 172, 180; Union of South Africa, 178
South African Army, 93
South African Communist Party (SACP), 47–48
South African diaspora, 12
South African National Museum, 13
South African National Student Congress, 180–181
South African Nursing Council, 164
South African Republic (1881–1902), 109
South African Women's Federation (SAVF), 139
Southwest Africa (Namibia), 93
staff meetings, 34–38
"state capture," 82. *See also* corruption discourses
statues, 47–48, 117
stereotypes, as reference point for self-definition, 3–4, 189–190
Steyn, J. C., 168
Steyn, Melissa, 63–66
subdivisions, 139–140
Suid-Afrikaanse Vroue Federasie (SAVF), 139
superego, x
Surplus People, The (Platzky and Walker), 27
Suzan Kruger (ship), 166

INDEX 221

Suzman, Helen, 168
Suzman, Janet, 15
Swati (Swazi) people, 35, 113. *See also* eSwatini, Kingdom of

Tabuchi, Antonio, 89
Tambo, Oliver, 172, 173; O. R. Tambo International Airport, 53
tax, black, 140, 162
technology, 35, 62–63, 124
testimony, 4. *See also* confessions
Themba (public hospital), 31, 38, 72
Theron, Charlize, 111
Thompson, Jarred, 2
Thulare, Daniel Mafeleu, 13
Till, Emmett, 13
touch, 53–54, 61
townships, 15, 31, 43; black people's relocation to, 5, 142; "location" as term for, 102. *See also* "homelands"; Mahushu (town)
transitions, 7, 12, 26, 147, 190
trauma, 2, 83, 100; and memories, 172–173
travel (agency) nurses, 83–84, 107. *See also* nurses
Truth and Reconciliation Commission, 172, 180
Tswana people, 122. *See also* Botswana; Bechuanaland
Tutu, Desmond, 26, 55

ubuntu (showing humanity), 77, 140–141, 162
ukwakumkanya (shadowed perspective), 28, 205n16
Umkhonto weSizwe (former military wing of ANC), 191
umphako (food taken on a journey), 5
un-becoming, 189, 213n15. *See also* dis-identification
United States, 20; aging prison population, 202n23; baby boomers, 10, 14, 49, 83; black domestic workers in storylines, 16; Confederate flag, 47; health insurance, 7; imagined racial population-demographic shift, 14; Ku Klux Klan, 126; lack of protections from discrimination, 25; long-term care, 10, 20; medical record-keeping systems, 35; racism faced by elder care workers, 78; real estate practice, 140; Republican Party, 22; senior housing, 60; Social Security, 22, 61; violence, 58, 60, 82; "witches," 97

van der Westhuizen, Christi, 131
van Riebeeck, Jan, 112–113, 115
van Wyk, Ilana, 132
vendors, at grant queues, 23
violence, 58, 60, 82
Vlakplaas, 180–182

waiting, 22–23, 28, 90, 107, 125, 136, 182; for afterlife, 133–134
Waiting (Crapanzano), 14–15
waiting rooms, 6–7
Waluś, Janusz, 48
White, Luise, 119–120
"white genocide," 14
white nationalists, 13–14, 139, 187
Whiteness Just Isn't What It Used to Be: White Identity in a Changing South Africa (Steyn), 63
whiteness studies, 63, 131
white people: anxieties of, 8–9, 14, 113, 187; beliefs, Fox News-ification of, 13, 191; and stereotype of "old racists," 2–3, 17; white saviorism, 138
whites in South Africa: and banality, 14–15; poorer older, social welfare policy for, 10; white women, prerogative to uplift nation, 10
white supremacy, 9, 17, 106; and life expectancy disparities, 13–14
Wickware, Marvin E., Jr., 187
wildlife, 87–90, 122. *See also* elephants; *mabhalane* (secretary bird)
Willemse, Willie, 168
"witches" and witchfinders, 97–100, 105–106, 147; Salem, Massachusetts, 97
Wolff, M., 191
Woman Next Door, The (Omotoso), 16
Woolworth's, 41
World Vision, 68

X (formerly Twitter), 13, 113, 203n24

"Yesterday is history, tomorrow is a mystery" saying, 45, 46, 126, 191
youth movements. *See* Comrades (youth group); generations: contrasts between

Zimbabwe, 116–123. *See also* Rhodesia (Zimbabwe)
Zimbabwean War of Liberation, 47, 116–119
Zion Church in Christ (ZCC), 101
Zuma, Jacob, 48, 81

About the Author

Casey Golomski is an award-winning creative writer and cultural and medical anthropologist, centering perennial questions about life, death, and their thresholds to ask how we work through and commemorate critical events in our lives and communities. He is an associate professor of anthropology and women's and gender studies at the University of New Hampshire in Durham, New Hampshire, as well as a visiting researcher at Wits University in Johannesburg, and lives in Medford, Massachusetts. He is the author of many literary and academic works, including the book *Funeral Culture*, and has been interviewed for or cited by the *New York Times*, New Hampshire Public Radio, *New Hampshire Magazine*, *Alex News*, *Times of Eswatini*, and *Business Times*.